"I do not pretend that I ha[ve never done wrong, but no] one fault justifies another, bu[t nevertheless, those who judge] like mine should remember th[at the darkest life may have a] bright side, and that after the wor[st has been said against a] man, he may, if he is heard, tell a story in his own rough way that will perhaps lead them to intimate the harshness of their thoughts against him, and find as many excuses for him as he would plead for himself."

Ned Kelly – bushranger
The Age
August 9, 1880

BLACK

By Heath Black with Lisa Holland-McNair

agendaPUBLISHING

Published by Agenda Publishing www.agendapublishing.com.au

First published in 2012

Copyright © Heath Black and Lisa Holland-McNair 2012

The moral rights of the authors have been asserted.

All rights reserved. No part of this book may be reproduced or transmitted by any person or entity (including Google, Amazon or similar organisation), in any form or by any means, electronic or mechanical, including photocopying, recording, scanning or by any information storage and retrieval system, without prior permission in writing from the authors. The Australian *Copyright Act 1968* (the Act) allows a maximum of one chapter or 10 per cent of this book, whichever is the greater, to be photocopied by any educational institution for its educational purposes provided that the educational institution (or body that administers it) has given a remuneration notice to Copyright Agency Limited (CAL) under the Act.

National Library of Australia
Cataloguing-in-Publications entry:

Black, Heath, 1979–
Black / by Heath Black with Lisa Holland-McNair.

ISBN: 9780987132307 (pbk.)

Black, Heath.
Australian football players--Biography.
Football players--Australia--Biography.
Manic-depressive illness--Australia--Biography.
Attention-deficit disorder in adults--Australia--Biography.

Other Authors/Contributors: Holland-McNair, Lisa, 1970–

796.336092

Cover photography: Daniel Wilkins, STM
Cover design: Keely Barrow, Inspire2Design
Editor: Jan Hallam
Designer: Platform Communications
Printing: Scott Print

www.heathblack.com.au

ACKNOWLEDGMENTS

Writing and publishing this book has been a strange, intriguing and ultimately fulfilling journey made possible by the help and support of an unusual, and talented, collection of people.

We express our sincere thanks and gratitude to the following people: Barbara Holland who transcribed hour upon hour of raw interviews, Jan Hallam our editor who tidied and tightened for us, Kerry Harmanis our benefactor who made it possible for us to publish the book ourselves, our legal team John Prior and Jason MacLaurin who gave us their professional advice unconditionally, Dr John Clarkson who generously provided us with his expert opinion, Gary Bryant who helped us get back on track with his support, Sonia Nolan our proof-reader extraordinaire, Keely Barrow from Inspire2Design for her edgy cover design, Kirsty Danby and the team at Platform Communications for their great marketing support, and the Fremantle Dockers, in particular Steve Roscich, who helped ensure the book reached as many people as possible. A big thank you also to the Mecca Chicks – Tania Hudson, Sonia Nolan, Kylie Ashenbrenner, Sonia Miller and Corinne Hawke – who read numerous edits and provided valuable and constructive advice and support.

Thank you to Heath and Asha's families for supporting them both in their decision to publish such a raw and confronting retelling of their lives.

Finally, thank you to our partners Asha and Dean for all their help, support and patience during the past three years.

Heath Black and Lisa Holland-McNair

A percentage of the profits of the sales of *Black* will be donated to the Men's Advisory Network (MAN) www.man.org.au

CONTENTS

Introduction vii
Prologue by Heath Black xi
A Note from the Author.. xiii

Chapter 1	Rock Bottom 1
Chapter 2	The Guillotine Falls 13
Chapter 3	Rebel with a Reason 23
Chapter 4	So the Sacrifice Begins 31
Chapter 5	Dreams Come True 41
Chapter 6	Welcome to the AFL 53
Chapter 7	Fear and Loathing 67
Chapter 8	A Losing Streak at the Gallops 75
Chapter 9	The Demon Drink 83
Chapter 10	The Light at the End 91
Chapter 11	Ring of Fire 99
Chapter 12	Through the Eyes of a Loved One by Asha Montgomerie 113

Epilogue by Lisa Holland-McNair 129

INTRODUCTION

Since the very first game of Australian Rules Football some 150 years ago, young men have battled it out on the football field, playing one of the world's toughest team sports. The Victorian Football League (VFL) was the stronghold for football until it expanded to a national competition in the late 1980s. In 1990 it officially became the Australian Football League, or the AFL as it is better known.

Fans as a result were presented with a tough choice: stick with their original VFL team or switch allegiances and support their new local team.

An interesting phenomenon arose following the creation of the teams in states outside of Victoria. The Victorian fans were used to seeing footy players living their lives around the suburbs and, in typical Australian style, usually admired them from afar. In Perth it was a different story. The West Australian Football League (WAFL) players certainly had their fair share of fans, but AFL footballers were few and far between, so spotting one, especially the higher profile players, was usually accompanied by a request for an autograph or in more ugly circumstances, a drunken approach for a fight.

The West Coast Eagles bore the brunt of this for many years, their fans, the media and public alike putting them on pedestals and treating them as celebrities. Many young boys wanted to be a footballer and many young girls dreamt of being a footballer's girlfriend, or WAG (Wives And Girlfriends), as they now are known.

INTRODUCTION

Some AFL players were able to handle the attention well, presenting as solid role models for youngsters. Others struggled and the public started to see more and more newspaper reports of drunken fights, sex scandals and arrests.

Their fans forgave them. In most cases the clubs and the AFL also forgave them, either through some enforced time off or a transfer to another club. On the field players were celebrated for their toughness and how hard they could play and these qualities were sought after by recruiters and encouraged by coaches. This was what the game was about – a game for hard men.

One such footballer was Heath Black. Heath played for Fremantle and St Kilda as a midfielder for 12 years, notching up almost 200 AFL games. He was known on the field as a tough competitor, often matching up with other hard men. He joined a fledging Fremantle Dockers' side in just its second year in the league, as a Victorian draftee along with fellow Vic Jess Sinclair. They were fairly unique creatures to come West to play and from the moment they landed on Sandgroper soil, the media wanted a piece of them.

Heath made a solid start to his football career. He played his first AFL game in Round 4 of his first year with the Dockers. The 18-year-old, fast-footed lefty quickly became an important part of the team, and later received a tidy sum to move back home to Victoria to join St Kilda. Family commitments prompted him to return to the West and to the Dockers, but soon after his return, things started going awry.

INTRODUCTION

On New Year's Day in 2006 he found himself in trouble at Perth Cup celebrations at Ascot Racecourse resulting in him being prosecuted for a series of offences. Later that year he was charged for disorderly conduct when he was arrested for urinating in public. He announced his retirement from the AFL at the end of 2008, but stayed involved in football, signing up to play for WAFL club Peel Thunder in January 2009.

Injury and a lost passion for the game prompted him to retire from football a few months later, walking away from Peel and starting work as a media commentator at Channel 7. But trouble wasn't far away. Following the breakdown of his marriage, Heath once again found himself in strife with the police in July, this time pleading guilty to disorderly conduct after an incident outside a nightclub in Northbridge, on the fringe of Perth's CBD. This was quickly followed by another similar charge in September when he got into a fight in a North Perth bar. A couple of weeks later, police found Heath asleep in his car, after running into a kerb. He was charged with drink-driving.

Many people struggle to understand the problem with these men. Why can't they control themselves and just walk away from trouble? What factors contribute to their troubled lives? Is it the money? Is it the fame? Is it the lifestyle?

For Heath, many of his problems stemmed from alcohol abuse, mental health issues and anxiety created from pressures he experienced from fans both on and off the field, women drawn to celebrity and prowess of an

INTRODUCTION

alpha male, and what to do with his life when his football career had already peaked.

But it's not all about the football.

Like most boys of his generation and before, Heath was raised to be tough and grow into a 'blokey bloke'. This contributed to his lack of awareness about his growing mental instability, and impeded his ability to ask for help. This is not unusual in our Australian society where men are told to 'toughen up' or 'grow a backbone'. Times are changing, but still there are many men who don't have a good support network or feel they can't speak out about their feelings or the things which are troubling them.

For our boys and our future generations this has to change.

PROLOGUE

I started this book nearly three years ago in June 2009, not long after I walked away from the great game of Australian Rules Football. Since leaving the game things have not come so easy. I've been arrested, abused, assaulted and gone through an ugly divorce. My pre-existing anxiety and Bipolar II have spiralled out of control and I've used alcohol to drown my sorrows.

My life really was a mess and I feel by sharing my story I might be able to provide some insight to others who may be looking to walk in my footy boots, or those who wake up in the morning thinking life just feels a bit too hard.

Aussie Rules is a great game and I will be eternally grateful to have played at the top level for 12 years. But there are so many deeper issues which crop up when you are at the top of your game: the anxiety, the expectation of fans, on and off the field, the drugs and alcohol and finally the fallout when you're spat out the other end.

Of course, many of these issues are not exclusive to footy. I bet there are people, men in particular, from all walks of life, who can relate to these issues. Whether it's kicking a footy in the AFL, driving a tank in the Army, repairing a 400 tonne dump truck, shearing a sheep or picking up a pen at the office, sometimes life can go completely off the tracks. You wake up one day and wonder how you got so far off course.

PROLOGUE

So why listen to Blacky telling you these things, and why now? Footy has been the centre of my life since I was 12, but I was suddenly faced with an uncertain future and a whole heap of shit I needed to sort through. Even though for me it came down to misdiagnosis of a mental illness, I believe this type of life crisis is much more widespread than we care to admit.

If you're living a life where you just don't seem to be able to get on track, I hope something in my story starts those alarm bells ringing. There's help out there, you just need to ask.

Heath Black, 2012

A NOTE FROM THE AUTHOR

I have been interviewing Heath and writing *Black* since July 2009.

During the three year time period between starting the book and finally releasing it in April 2012, Heath's life and state of mind have soared and plunged, careening along a very erratic path.

This journey is reflected in the tone and style of the book.

The first nine chapters are predominantly based on interviews in 2009, a time Heath was misdiagnosed, on the wrong medication and at the height of his manic behaviour. Chapter 10 was written in early-2011 after Heath had spent the past year getting his life back on track and when he was diagnosed with Bipolar II.

The final chapter of *Black* – Ring of Fire – was only written in December 2011, after Heath received confirmation he also had Adult ADHD and as he was preparing to start his new life with Asha in Victoria.

As a result of this, some readers may find contradictions or repetition in the book. We have decided not to edit these out, and feel that by staying true to Heath's state of mind, readers can truly experience the roller coaster journey which has been Heath's life, and is often the life of people with mental illness.

Lisa Holland-McNair

CHAPTER 1
ROCK BOTTOM

"I'm not proud of it, in fact it is the most shameful thing I have ever done, but today I feel I need to be honest about the monster I had become, look it in the eye and stare it down."

What is it about finally hitting rock bottom? No job, no colleagues and no real friends. It's like you've gone from being Superman where everything you touch turns to gold, to everything, and everyone, you touch turning to shit. You look around and it seems everyone who was ever in your life has just packed up and gone, leaving you alone to pick up the pieces.

And you know what? Although it doesn't help, you can't blame them: you can only blame yourself.

I had begun my descent down a very slippery slope in the lead-up to my retirement from the AFL. I managed to control that slide to a degree while I was still playing, but once I had retired, I started free-falling.

The true manic episodes started on my final footy trip to Thailand in August 2008, which I write about later in the book. However, by 2009, the extreme behaviour was occurring on a regular basis. On a private trip to Bali I got involved in an incident and lost the plot to the point where I think I very nearly killed a bloke.

The whole event is a blur because I was in such a blind rage and totally consumed with paranoia. The only way I can recall what happened is through the eyes of my brother, who was there at the time.

I'm not proud of it, in fact it is the most shameful thing I have ever done, but today I feel I need to reflect on this incident; to be honest about the monster I had become, look it in the eye and stare it down. Talking about it goes some way towards beating it.

I had gone to Bali with my then-girlfriend and now wife Asha, my younger brother Shaun and his ex-girlfriend, Alex. Let's not bullshit here, by this stage I already was the monster, and this trip was my opportunity to let the beast roam free. I was no longer under the constraints of the AFL and I was away from the prying eyes of Perth. I had every intention of taking it all up a few notches. Yeah, I'd had a gun pulled on me in Thailand, but I wondered if I could go one step further. Did I care that Asha was with me? No fucking way; all I cared about was feeding the monster inside.

Alcohol was my drug of choice and I don't think I went anywhere in Bali without a beer firmly clasped in my hand. We'd go out at night; I'd get smashed, drop into bed at 4am, wake up at 7am and grab another beer. I was constantly drunk and as a result I was constantly anxious and getting more and more paranoid.

ROCK BOTTOM

My brother Shaun is a great guy. He's nine years younger than me so he was only 18 at the time we were in Bali. He's a small guy too, shorter than me and weighed about 70kg back then. One night the four of us went out to this nightclub we'd been to several times before and Shaun and I had our shirts off, drinking and having a good time. Next thing I knew I felt liquid running down my bare back and I knew someone had spat alcohol on me from a straw. I turned around expecting to see some young buck wanting to have a go but I was shocked to find the guy who'd done it was an elderly, fat dude, standing there with a bunch of other elderly blokes.

This guy just looks at me and declares *"I am Russian"*. Now this may sound like something out of a David Lynch film, but suddenly my pulse rate went through the roof and I immediately switched on to full alert. A good friend of mine had warned me that there were a lot of Russian underworld figures hanging out in Bali and to just 'be aware'.

Nothing actually happened with these blokes, but my already hyper state clicked up a notch to fuel the rage and increase my paranoia. Because I hadn't been diagnosed properly I wasn't aware that I was having a full-on paranoid episode.

Asha and Alex left the nightclub to go back to our hotel and Shaun and I decided to keep partying on. With every bar or nightclub we went to, I felt there were Russians watching, ready to attack me or my brother. Finally at about 6am when I had drunk myself almost sober, we were walking back to our hotel. It was pouring with rain, the streets were flooded and we were off our faces, wrestling and skylarking around. We were walking down this dark alley in a very seedy part of Bali when these two guys on a scooter rode past. Just as they passed I jumped in a puddle splashing them, which was a bit of fun, but a real dickhead thing to do. The guys were saturated from the rain anyway, but did they keep riding? No, the stupid idiots turned around and came back, got off the bike, opened their mouths and, yep, they turn out to be Russian.

I can honestly say I don't recall what happened next because I went into a full-on blind rage.

I have experienced this type of thing previously on the footy field. You come off the ground after being reported for an incident and the coach says *"did you hit him?"* and you say *"no, no"* and then you look on the video and sure enough, you've gone smack. That's blind rage because you just can't remember doing it. I did that a lot in football, probably twice a year. I have always had anger issues, it's just that footy let me use it rather than punish me for it.

In footy the consequence of your actions is simple: suspension for a couple of weeks. Sure you have let the team down, you go back to your club, the coach rings you, he calls you a bloody idiot, you need to address your anger and the coach doesn't talk to you for a couple of weeks, that's about the extent of it. You also then get physically flogged in training. I was in front of the Tribunal about 11 times in my career, more often than not I got caught. You get a reputation for that sort of thing and I think the umpires look out for it.

ROCK BOTTOM

When I played, my coaches always told us to go to the absolute edge of being reported but don't cross that line. You are encouraged in every way to intimidate, to overpower, and to do anything you can to get your player off his guard. Don't get me wrong, I doubt that my ability to lose my temper was seen as a plus for the game. I think it was totally negative for my team because the opposition would know that I was a ticking time bomb and they would come at me and say stuff to throw me off. I was a liability in that sense, but maybe for both the Dockers and the Saints the positives outweighed the negatives. In playing and setting up goals, this explosion of anger would happen and it would certainly pay off more times than not.

I couldn't fix it, but more to the point, I didn't really want to fix it and I didn't care. It would probably have been beneficial to target someone I could talk to back then, when all these protocols and support mechanisms were in place; certainly from a club point of view they would tick every box to help me, but was that going to change me? No, it wasn't. I was an extreme case, but hell, there are lots of extreme cases in the AFL.

Looking back, I realise that if I didn't have football to pull me back into line a fair bit, I don't know what the hell would've happened to me. I probably would've been in jail for a start, and I suppose I have to be pretty thankful for football keeping me on track... to a point that is.

Getting back to the Russians. It has been only recently that I have spoken to Shaun about what really happened that night and he has been able to get this huge burden off his chest, which he's been carrying around with him all this time.

The Russians got off their bike and asked me why I'd splashed them, nothing more than that at this point. But for me the Russian accent was all I heard and I just wanted to kill them. It was that simple. I wanted to protect my brother and I thought I just had to kill them before they killed us.

I walked straight up to one guy but he was already on the front foot and head butted me with his helmet on. I was knocked down and my nose was splattered across my face and, you know what? I just thought 'good, it's open slather'.

I punched him but missed his face and copped his helmet, injuring my hand. Not that it mattered. I went again and with one punch straight in the face knocked him down and out. I then walked up to his mate, who had his arms up and was backing away, but I just started to punch him again and again in the face. Punch after punch … I was turning his face into a bloody pulp and even after my brother jumped on my back to try and stop me I kept going. He said it was like he wasn't even there and I was making these weird sounds, a bit like a bull snorting.

I finally stopped hitting the guy but I still hadn't finished. I picked up their scooter with some kind of super human strength - the rage was so strong - and just slammed it into the ground; again and again and again. The exhaust pipe was burning into my forearm but I didn't feel it.

My brother finally got me out of there and we turned up at the hotel. I was bleeding and my hand was puffed up like a tennis ball. I was still fired up though, grunting like a bull and contemplating going out and getting some more action. It wasn't until the next day when I'd slept and sobered up that I calmed down. But then my anxiety kicked in – were the Balinese police going to turn up, or the Russian mafia? I was bedridden for a day and a half with constant diarrhoea, crippled by the anxiety.

I wasn't physically sick, I was just sick in the head. A big part of me actually thought the best place for me was rotting away in a stinking Bali prison.

Of course all of this was overseas, away from most of my family, friends and work colleagues.

The face of my monster was finally seen in Australia about half way through 2009, around the time I got into several fights in Perth and was arrested for drink-driving … again. It was nearly 12 months to the day since I'd announced my retirement from AFL.

FIGHTING IN NORTHBRIDGE

I look back now and realise that there were a lot of events which led to me losing control completely, but it all seemed to become very public after a misunderstanding outside a Northbridge nightclub in July 2009.

I had been attending courses and counselling for my alcohol abuse and anger management for years, and standing outside that nightclub in Northbridge that night I should have known better. I'd learnt that if something was making me uncomfortable, I had to tell myself to stop and go through a breathing pattern of 5, 4, 3, 2, 1; calm down and then just walk away. That is what I should have done at the nightclub when that guy was giving me shit. It bloody works, but you need to practise it three or four times a day.

The other thing that helps me calm down is to have a long shower or a hot bath - just to have water on my body. If I don't do that, I start to get sloppy, and shit like Northbridge happens. It's like anything in life, though, if things are going along all right you think you no longer need to maintain them. You forget that what got you to that positive place, and what keeps you there, is all the hard work.

Back to Northbridge, I don't know why I couldn't walk away when the guy was giving me shit. It wasn't like it was a huge fight or anything; I didn't even punch him, I just kind of wrestled him to the ground, but sure enough the coppers rounded me up and took me to the police lock-up. That's routine stuff in Perth's nightclub district of Northbridge. Once you get taken off the street for a violent incident, you get fully processed. The garage door goes up, the van drives in, the garage door comes down, the lock-up doors open and you are ditched straight into a viewing cell.

I had a big hoodie on so I just covered my head. There were other criminals in there but no cameras, which was one good thing. I was there for ages, about six hours in total, and I had to submit to a full strip search: so I had to pull the ball bag up, split the cheeks and cough. When you get released from the lock-up, it's like it is in the movies, I'm not kidding. The garage door opens, you're on the street and you look left and then right. All I thought was 'where am I?' I had no idea so I ended up walking to Albany Highway. Finally, I jumped in a cab and got home at 6am. When I got home, I knew

Asha would not be happy, so I tapped on the door and just passed her all the paperwork telling her I'd been locked up. At least then she knew I wasn't cheating on her.

HYDE PARK HOTEL

The alarm bells started to ring then, but not quite loud enough because about eight weeks later, in late-September, I was involved in another incident at the Hyde Park Hotel in Perth.

This day I was in a really black mood. I used to go to the Hyde Park nearly every day while Asha was at work. I'd just sit at the bar, drinking beer. It was the middle of the day and there were four people at the bar and I was in a real shitty mood, just angry, probably on the back of a bender and lowered by a hangover. I was really anxious and really on edge, I was totally manic in a way. I had a lot of energy and I powered down a couple of really quick pints to settle that down. There was a guy in there who I thought was a drug dealer. I thought I had seen him sell drugs to kids. I had seen him there a lot and he had never bothered me before. If you are drinking at the Hyde Park you are mixing with some interesting and different people; I don't say different in a bad way because I was there and I am different. The Hyde Park Hotel was like a safe house for me.

What got to me this time was this guy started to ask me about my kids. It caused me to snap because in my mind, this guy was a drug dealer. I was clearly quite paranoid and making up stories in my own head. Before I knew it, a young barmaid was pushing me off the guy. When I saw she was scared I just got up and left. As I was leaving, the guy's missus touched my arm and then just dropped to the ground and appeared to faint. She wouldn't get up and they had to ring an ambulance. I just walked home, and on the way went to KFC to get a 21-piece bucket. None of it worried me at the time. I could see the ambulance coming, so I knew then that the cops would attend as that is a requirement when an ambulance is called in Northbridge. At this stage, I still believed that I had done the right thing by giving a drug dealer a bit of a touch-up.

I got home and sat down, this was about 6pm, and Asha was cooking dinner and I didn't say a word. Asha reckons I was sitting down and breathing quite heavily. She asked if I was all right, but I just sat there and didn't say a word. Later on the cops rang and asked if I had been involved in a fight at the Hyde Park. I said *"yes"*, and so they charged me with disorderly conduct and I had to pay a fine.

When I look back on this period, what's more important to me than the charges and fines, and what breaks my heart, is when I think about what Asha was putting up with. She isn't a violent person at all. I was going through a black stage and she was on that wild roller-coaster ride with me, and not knowing what was going through my head. I'm not saying that Asha and I fought, we didn't, we were extremely close, but I was living this other life that she struggled to understand. She would go to work and I would get pissed, she knew that, but the fighting and anger was increasing ... and increasing. My depression and anxiety were going through the roof.

Then my dog, Sarge, got killed, and that just added to the blackness. I loved that dog. I was spiralling out of control and hitting the booze really hard.

I knocked myself out once trying to jump a fence when I was drunk when I went to South Australia to visit Asha's family. I woke up in the dirt under a car at the Olympic Dam Footy Club. Later that year when Asha's parents came over to Perth to visit, I ended up in jail again on another drunk and disorderly charge for falling asleep in public. Not cool, especially when her parents were here.

Most people didn't see that side of me though. I still had a job and was putting up a fair show in front of people. I could bullshit my way through the situations where I had to, and then quickly exit, come home and crack a beer – then everything was back to normal for me. That's how it was actually going, which wasn't good.

At one point I even asked Asha to leave. I said *"I think you had better go, I am giving you the opportunity here. I think it is best if you leave because I am pretty bad baggage at the moment, and you're not only dragging a suitcase, you've got a ball and chain behind it as well."* That's how I felt after the Hyde Park fight. I don't know why she didn't leave me; she is a beautiful and kind person. It's fair to say, though, that at the time I thought if she did leave me, it would have made things easier – one less person to bullshit to.

Of course she stood by me through all of it, as did my parents and the Australian Football League Players' Association. They were all working together to find out what could be done to help me. But was I helping

BLACK

myself? No. I was intent on self-destruction. In my sane moments I thought it couldn't get much worse. I'd hit rock bottom. But of course, I hadn't. More trouble was just around the corner.

CHAPTER 2
THE GUILLOTINE FALLS

"I knew that, quite rightly, and particularly with everything else that had been going on, the courts would not take this offence lightly. And, you know what, neither should they have. Drink-driving is unacceptable. I could have killed someone."

I had become a social pariah. Fights, arrests, public drunkenness, I did it all and, what was worse, I was not repentant about anything I had done. I cared about hurting Asha, but towards blokes in general, I had no feelings or remorse.

Then came October and another drink-driving charge and with that I had used up all my free passes. What was left of anything remotely good in my world came crashing down around my ears.

ARRESTED AGAIN

I was having drinks with a friend at my old haunt, Moondyne Joe's, which is a carbon copy of the Hyde Park but in Fremantle. I had a strong feeling I was about to lose my job as a television reporter because of the incident at the Hyde Park, and I was asking my mate if he could get me some work. I'd only planned on having a couple of beers, but as I was about to wind things up one of my closest mates walked in and, lo and behold, it was his birthday. I rang Asha, telling her I was going to have to stay and I would get a taxi home.

Straight away we just got into it. It was a birthday celebration after all. I started drinking beer but then made a crucial mistake; I switched, which I never do, and went to vodka and lemonade. It went a bit hazy from there but I remember the alarm bells ringing and I knew it was time to go home. I snuck off without even saying goodbye to anyone and got in the car and drove off.

No one knew I was driving – they would have stopped me if they had. I stopped at a service station, got something to eat, and got back into the car and took off. I was trying to open the food package when I hit the kerb, popping the front and back tyres on to the rims. Through the drunken haze, I knew I was in a big steaming pile of shit.

I didn't have much time so I pulled the car up onto the verge, two wheels right up off the road. I rang Asha and I said, *"I've hit a kerb and I have popped the tyres. I have a mate who owns a tow truck who I'll call, it will cost me $80, I will take the keys out of the ignition, recline the chair and sleep it off."* I was adamant this wasn't her problem, so she shouldn't do anything. I didn't ring my tow truck mate because I went straight to sleep, still in the car. Someone else rang the cops when they saw this guy – me – slumped over the steering wheel. Three hours later, tap, tap, tap, and I was gone. Arrested again. Once more I had made a really bad mistake.

I'd already been done for drink-driving in October 2008, following the break-up of my marriage and after I had announced my retirement from the AFL. I knew that, quite rightly, and particularly with everything else that had been going on, the courts would not take this offence lightly. And, you know what, neither should they have. Drink-driving is unacceptable. I could have killed someone.

With the assault charges and now the drink-driving charge, my family was ready to intervene and the AFL Players Association (AFLPA) was fully involved, even though I had retired. The way it works is that for three years after retirement you are still under the umbrella of the AFLPA. Looking back, it was a mini intervention. My family wanted me to move back to Melbourne and booked a plane trip for me within 24 hours of the drink-driving charge. I didn't go. For God's sake, I was a 30-year-old man who had started to realise finally I had to deal with my own issues and sort out my own shit.

The AFLPA put me in contact with a doctor who works with elite athletes in Perth, including both Freo and West Coast players, in the areas of drug and alcohol abuse. We then began trying to work out what was wrong with me.

I spoke to the media about my depression and anxiety and met with the psychiatrist. By that stage I was really starting to question whether I was medicated properly. I had been on anti-depressants for a couple of years and they didn't seem to be working. However, I'd always had a fair share of alcohol in the mix. The question I wanted answered was what would happen when alcohol was taken away? It seems bloody obvious now, but it finally hit me that to get better the number one thing to address was my abuse of alcohol.

TACKLING ALCOHOL

The short-term answer to this, according to my shrink, was a tablet called Antabuse. The way it was explained to me was that when you take these tablets you can't have one drop of alcohol because it will make you violently ill.

I got on really well with my doctor and I knew I had to do something … but I wasn't willing to take these tablets. He told me fair and square I needed to prove to the courts, to my family, to everyone, that I was prepared to do something to fix my problems. In my head I knew it was the right thing to do, but a huge part of me didn't want to take them. After I read about all the potential side effects, my anxiety kicked in big time. I didn't know what the pill would do to me. One of the side effects is death and I even convinced myself I might die if I took it. The tablets are designed to react to any type of alcohol, not just alcohol you drink, but it could be Listerine, hand wash or cologne, anything alcohol-based. Those three things are part of my daily routine. It is such a weak feeling when you know what you should do to help yourself, but you just can't bring yourself to do it because you are scared.

So I never did take the pill.

Let's be completely honest here, it wasn't just the fear of side effects. Drinking still felt good, especially in moderation. I knew I couldn't drink to the point where I was intoxicated or going stupid, but I wanted to try to take control of myself and not have the tablet control me. My initial answer to it all was to not put myself in a situation where I could get into trouble again. All the brawls had been in or around pubs, and drink-driving is obviously linked to over consumption of booze. So I thought, I won't be in a pub, I won't be intoxicated in a public place; it's about risk management. I was also attending an alcohol-based program on Mondays and then every second Tuesday I did hypnotherapy and more counselling.

It took me a long time to realise that every time I have a drink of alcohol, one drop, that's a risk for me because of the way I respond to alcohol. For me alcohol creates depression. If I am bingeing my anxiety goes through the roof and it increases aggression. All the occasions I have been in trouble with the law have always had alcohol involved. I have never gotten into trouble when I've been sober – never ever. Nowadays I limit my drinking and I'm careful about where I drink. I know when I've had enough, I can feel that other part of me wanting to get out and do some damage. At those times I just stop drinking or go home.

GETTING THE SACK

It was during all this counselling and work to try and get me off the grog that I realised how much of a pariah I had become. After the drink-driving charge I was finally terminated from my job as a football commentator on Channel 7. It was a fair cop. They'd given me a fair go. They'd backed me during both the Northbridge and Hyde Park Hotel assaults. Channel 7 was the only media I spoke to after the Hyde Park incident. The day after the Hyde Park fight I got home from my morning at the gym and was in the kitchen. I looked out the front and couldn't believe my eyes – Channel 7, Channel 10, Channel 9, the ABC, they were all there, outside the unit. One of them told me the police media unit had let them know. That's how it is here in Perth.

I don't blame the media. I let the Channel 7 guys in because I worked with them. They wanted a comment but I wasn't going to make a comment on this one. I wasn't nervous about losing my job at this stage, which looking back doesn't make sense and shows just how delusional I had become. I thought I was invincible. It's all crazy, but I was blind to the implications of many of my actions. I really did love that job at Channel 7 and I threw it straight down the toilet.

If I thought the media interest after the Hyde Park incident was bad, it was nothing compared to the drink-driving incident on October 14.

THE GUILLOTINE FALLS

The media were camped out the front of my house for 48 hours after that one.

So here I was in late 2009. I had lost my job with Channel 7 and was awaiting several court hearings for the various charges. My other job at the time was in a private property development business. The guys in the business were both my partners and my mates. The drink-driving charge was also the final nail in the coffin for them, and they decided to pull the pin on me as well.

It was a fair enough call. From a business point of view I totally understand it. As one of them wrote in my termination email, which is I how I found out I was out on my arse, *"you can't defend the indefensible"*. I'd put them in a position where people would come up to them and say, *"what are you doing employing this guy? He is a liability, he is an alcoholic, he is a violent person"*.

The business point of view is one thing, but I was at the lowest point in my life and I counted these guys as my friends. I'd spent the past 12 months working with them on building up the business and then I was out with just an email. In a way, I understand that too. They had a lot invested in me and I had stuffed it up.

It hurt and was really hard to take because I am a proud and loyal man. But I felt like I was a bloody dickhead at the end of the day. I felt disappointed with myself. I lost an opportunity to develop a good career option outside of football. Looking back, I just wasn't ready and I still hadn't worked out what was wrong with me.

BIPOLAR II

My counsellor and I kept working at it – together and separately. It wasn't an easy journey to find the solution, but it turned out to be a fairly simple fix. In a nutshell we worked out that I didn't have the previously diagnosed depression, and instead established that it was Bipolar II. Bipolar II disorder happens when a person has episodes of both hypomania and depression, but no manic episodes.

Even though nearly every aspect of my life had turned to shit, when I was told it was Bipolar II it felt like a huge weight had been lifted off my shoulders. It was just a massive relief. I was walking out of my doctor's office an hour later with a script for a new medication called lithium and with high hopes that I could be normal. As 2009 turned into 2010, I found myself in Port Lincoln in South Australia with loved ones, getting off my old medication and on to the new stuff.

When it all crumbled, probably the number one thing that I got out of hitting rock bottom – well, it was actually worse than rock bottom – was that it was a clean slate for me. I sat back while the whole world was crumbling around me and I thought 'what am I going to do?' I was looking at nothing, so it was like I was able to start making decisions without reference to anything or anyone.

I had an opportunity to pick what I wanted to do, and I could only think of football. I asked myself, if I needed to leave Perth. I knew the answer was yes. I needed to get out of Perth because living in Northbridge made it too easy for me to end up in a pub and then get into trouble.

I needed to get back into footy, preferably in a community-oriented club, so I just started ringing people in the south west. I was probably the most unemployable person in Western Australia, but I just kept ringing and ringing and asked people to meet me so they could see that when I'm not drinking, I'm an OK kind of bloke. As my mum has always told me, *"you are one of the most amazing people, sober – caring, you've got it all. But you are an absolute arsehole when you are drunk."* Thanks Mum.

I love my parents dearly and they have certainly stood by me throughout the whole fuckup my life had become, but I was starting to question how my childhood might have impacted on who I'd turned out to be. It turns out that it was a worthwhile path to track back down.

BLACK

CHAPTER 3
REBEL WITH A REASON

> "After retiring from professional football, I suppose I just slipped back into that full-on rebellion against society in general. Sort of what I had growing up – good, rebel, good, rebel and so on."

To understand where I am now, I need to go back to where it all started and how football shaped my life. I'm not a Sandgroper, although lots of people think I am. I was born and raised in Victoria, in Melbourne's eastern suburbs.

GROWING UP

It was 1979 and I was the only child of my Mum, Michele, and my Dad, Russell. Dad and Mum were born and bred in the knock-about Melbourne suburb of Ashburton. They grew up there, fell in love at a very young age and had me. Mum was a homemaker and Dad was a garbo. Back then we lived in Montrose – or Twinkle Town as the locals called it – which is about 40 kilometres east of Melbourne at the base of the Dandenong Ranges. Twinkle Town had a strong sense of community, a big obsession with sport and its own football team.

When my folks were together, life at home was volatile and not a very happy place for a kid to be. Dad drank and Mum wasn't prepared to put up with it, so Mum's parents were always urging her to leave. She never has been a big drinker and would always tell Dad what she thought, which usually ended up with holes in the walls and that sort of stuff. I suppose it still haunts me a bit, and although it shames me to admit it, I did find myself repeating that sort of pattern later in life; losing my temper, punching walls and doors, carrying on like a right dickhead and intimidating my ex-wife. The sort of stuff which is just totally unacceptable. Don't get me wrong, I'm not blaming my parents, I take full responsibility for my actions. I'm also not saying that my parents didn't look after me, they did, but it wasn't the best environment for a young child to grow up in.

Mum finally packed up and left Dad when I was three, taking me to stay with relatives in Queensland. The divorce wasn't consensual – at the time Dad really wanted Mum to stay, but Mum had to escape. We eventually moved back to Victoria to live with Mum's parents. The bond I developed with Mum during that time was extremely strong; we were more like brother and sister, sharing a room with two single beds in her parent's house. She was so young, and we just kind of hung out together.

REBEL WITH A REASON

When I was four, Mum started dating Paul, a local boy who played football with Dad at Ashburton. He was a bit older than Dad, so although they knew each other, they didn't hang out together. Mum ended up marrying Paul and after a couple of moves, we settled down as a family in Mulgrave. I can't speak highly enough of Paul. He turned out to be a strong father figure, mentor, boss and my original football coach, all rolled into one. He was patient, calm, family-oriented and devoted to my mother. To be honest the way he embraced me, even though I was a complete little shit at the time, was admirable.

Mulgrave at the time was a fairly large middle-class suburb. I went to a little Catholic school called Good Shepherd Primary and then on to an all-boys high school called Mazenod College. I had lots of mates growing up and I'm still friends with many of them today. School didn't tickle my fancy at all; these days I'm sure I would have been diagnosed with ADHD* or something like that. I was all over the shop. Even now I struggle to sit still for more than an hour, although I am getting better. It's probably been only the last couple of years that I've been able to sit on a couch and watch a movie. All the psychologists I've seen say I'm too wired; I plan too many things in one day and if I don't tick them all off, it affects me.

Mum likes to claim credit for teaching me footy; it was quite different in the late '80s/early '90s to what it's like now. There was no such thing as Auskick and kids didn't start playing seriously until they were nine years old. Growing up with football was perfect for a kid like me, especially

---
* Heath was diagnosed with Adult ADHD in 2011.

with my determination and abundance of energy. I was an extremely single-minded only child, who by a very early age knew how to cope with being on my own. When I was growing up, Mum and Dad shared custody of me, so I spent a lot of time with both my real Dad and my step-Dad, who both loved football.

A lot of credit for my football success needs to go to Dad. He was a good footballer and made it to Hawthorn's Under-19s list. He was well known around our area and could play any position on the ground, a bit like I could. He was a hard sort of man, with a beautiful kick and was touted at the time as a VFL player. It never happened though because alcohol and camaraderie with his friends took over, and when he was given an ultimatum to change his lifestyle or miss out on top-grade football, he chose his lifestyle. To this day I think he regretted that decision. But he was always really involved with my football, both as a child and when I became a professional footballer. I think he saw what might have been his, although he never said that to me.

TWO DIFFERENT LIVES

Life for me was one of contrasts – life with Mum and Paul in Mulgrave and with Dad and Jan in Montrose. From Monday to Friday with Mum, I was a good Catholic boy who occasionally stuffed up at school; just a normal kid. Then Dad would pick me up and take the shackles off and we'd go back to Twinkle Town – it was more like having a big brother. We would spend many weekends at Warburton Airstrip riding trail bikes, or off ferreting and other fun stuff like that. Dad often hung around people younger than himself, who treated him a bit like an elder. It was their respect for him which sent me the message that his behaviour was acceptable, but looking back we got up to lots of things that weren't really normal for a child. There were times when Dad would pick me up on a Friday night and VB cans would be rolling around the car. We would, more often than not, end up at the Bayswater Hotel.

A lot of our time together, Dad would be drinking with his mates at parties, leaving me to my own devices, although always under someone's watchful eye. These guys put me under their wing, but sometimes their idea of right and wrong was a little blurred. Half the problem with Dad was, like me, he can't handle too much grog. It brings out an ugly side of us. Dad is a black-and-white type of guy. He's intelligent, street smart, and loves his friends. He's always been the patriarch. But he's also a worrier and I reckon he might suffer from anxiety too. Let's face it, there are not too many answers at the bottom of a beer bottle, especially when it ends up with someone getting hurt. All that said, Dad is the first person there to support me when the shit hits the fan, and when everyone else is ready to drop me. He always stands by me.

Looking back, I think I received a lot of mixed messages as a child. In certain situations now, when I am confronted with violence, I will go down that violent path rather than walk away. Growing up I would see grown men fighting to the point of unconsciousness; I would see people with guns; things a young child and teenager shouldn't see. Dad had a controlling nature and that rubbed off on me. It's really only in the past couple of years that I've tried to better manage my need for control.

TAKING CONTROL

Control really is a double-edged sword – it can work in your favour and it can go completely against you. The control of AFL football made it a good career choice for me. It's a lot like the military. You're told what to eat, when to sleep, whether you can or can't go out. You name it, you're told it. And, like the military, you dedicate the best years of your life to something that can never be a full-life career. You don't think of this when you're young and getting into it.

Control in footy, which really is lack of any individual control, suited my often-hyper personality. It gave me an outlet but I found it increasingly hard to manage the control issue off the field in my everyday life. Because I had no individual control in my work, I would go home to whoever my partner was at the time and try and reclaim some control. Obviously that posed a lot of problems with almost all my relationships, apart from Asha, having failed. It's taken a lot of counselling and hypnotherapy to try to curb that nature and I've slipped a few times. Of course, now that I'm on the right medication, it has helped a lot but that has been only a recent development.

I have always had a rebellious streak in me. It probably started way back when my parents split. When I was with Dad, he took the shackles off and the little rebel was free, but when I was back with Mum, she'd rein me in. But the thing is, I love that rebel part of me; being on the edge. Don't get me wrong, I wouldn't go and do something because I wanted to get into trouble, that's not true. It's just that the consequences were always secondary to the action, and it's hard to let that go.

When I turned 17 I was drafted into the AFL. All of a sudden I was told what to eat, not to drink, don't do this, don't do that. It was like walking a tightrope for 12 years. But I welcomed the control, toed the line and played the game. It was only after the game, I'd lose all control, down 20 beers and get smashed then go pissed to training the next day. That's how I managed to keep up my rebellious behaviour, even within the constraints of top level football.

People sometimes wonder how I got away with it. Who knows really, but my take on it is maybe the clubs put up with my behaviour because I was playing well, and they turned a blind eye to what was going on off the footy field. From what I could see it seemed to work that way throughout the league. Look at some of the players who seem to have got away with everything. It really depends on who you are, what sort of contract you have and having mates within the club. The game has changed now, I believe, especially with all the bad press some players, including me, have had over the years. It's also becoming a tougher game leaving way less room for rebellious behaviour.

After retiring from professional football, I suppose I just slipped back into that full-on rebellion against society in general. Sort of what I had growing up – good, rebel, good, rebel and so on. When I look back now there were so many things that shaped me and played a role in my slide – growing up in a split family, starting footy from such a young age, my hyperactivity, which most likely was the beginning of my mental illness. All these things contributed to that character the footy fans called Blacky.

In late 2008, as I was contemplating my retirement from footy, my marriage fell apart and I was kicked out of home. In fact, during the last few months I was playing in the AFL, I was living out of my car – literally eating and sleeping in my car. Unbelievably, I thought I was coping, but looking back it was all a charade.

I was actually contracted to play in 2009 but I just couldn't face it. Physically, I probably would have struggled, I might have had about 15 games still in me, but it was more mental for me. I was already in full-on destruction mode and knew I would have let the club down, let the coaches down, and let my teammates down. I would have got reported more often than not because I was becoming too aggressive on the field, and I would have kept drinking.

I would have done everything I wasn't meant to do because I didn't give a fuck about anything.

How had I got to this place? Where had that optimistic, determined little kid who loved footy above all things, gone?

CHAPTER 4
SO THE SACRIFICE BEGINS

"Looking back it's remarkable - not one 18th birthday party, not one 21st party. Even my own 21st was put back six months because I was playing footy and couldn't attend."

Growing up I played for a local football club called North Vale Junior Football Club - we wore Swans' colours – red and white. A lot of my friends played for Mazenod in the same competition. Back then footy was all about having fun with your friends and that's how it should be today. For me, closely linked to the fun was letting off a bit of steam, in terms of energy and anger. It was important for me to play a sport where I could by physical.

I used to get pulled up for being too rough when I was a young kid, and now I see kids in Auskick who remind me of what I was like. Kids get punished for being physical at that age because they're playing well above their years. They're hurting these other poor little kids. You can see the parents of the injured kids cringe. As for the parents of the rough kids, what can you do? You can't tell your kid to pull up if that is the natural way they play. I think you have to leave it up to the umpire's discretion to control the game; it isn't up to the parents. Parents behaving badly on the sidelines at junior football make me sick.

Back to my junior days. North Vale was unfortunately a shocking team and we were at the bottom of the ladder. By the time I reached the Under-13s side, the team was abandoned because there were not enough children. So I had a crucial decision to make. I was the youngest of all my friends as well as being one of the smallest. I was a really skinny little boy and also anaemic at one stage. I was often sick because I didn't eat properly, I was so hyped up. I was just too busy to eat, and when I did, I had a disgusting diet.

I had to decide: do I play with my friends who were on Mazenod, my school's team and an older team, or do I stay in my age group and play for the Panthers? My mum ended up making the decision for me because I was so small. I became a Panther. Unfortunately for my friends, Mazenod, was not very good. We were 12 years old and it mattered at that age if you were beaten by 10 goals and only won once a year. In terms of picking a winning side, Mum certainly made the right decision because the Panthers then were a great team. I like to win and even back then I was competitive. I played with the Panthers until I was 13 and we ended up playing in the grand final, but lost.

It was great to be in a top team but, looking back, I think Mum made the wrong decision; I should have stayed with my friends and had fun. They were on the bottom of

SO THE SACRIFICE BEGINS

the ladder, but, so what? Instead I was in a good team that was very successful, but I didn't have as much fun, and at that age it should be all about having fun. Once you get to the elite level, the day you walk through the door of an AFL footy club, the fun stops. So I say to all those youngsters: make the most of it and have some fun while you're young.

Instead of being driven by fun, I had an extreme determination to succeed. What I didn't know then, but know now, was that even at a young age I was always trying to prove something to my parents. They would hate me for saying it but I felt then, and now, I was never good enough. This came more from Mum than Dad. I remember when I was playing for the Dockers, I played a game at Subiaco when I was going through a really good patch. I might have had 35 touches but I didn't kick a goal because I was playing in the backline. I rang Mum and the first thing she said was *"why didn't you kick a goal? You should have done better"*. That's despite being named best-on-ground by a street.

She just never gave credit. When I asked her about this, she told me she was harsh on me so I wouldn't get a big head. I'd say *"Mum I'm 25 years old, I've been in the game for eight years, I'm not going to get a big head"*. All players know whether they have played a good or bad game and I was brutally honest with myself and my assessment of my games. I get why Mum was being harsh, but it would have been great once in a while to have a pat on the back from the people who meant the most to me.

Compliments sometimes did happen, but the negatives were always brought forward first; almost as a condition of the praise. After Mum's comments, I would ring Dad and he would be like, *"when are you going to win the Brownlow?"*. I led the poll one year, which was a bit of a joke. Even if I was playing really well, I'd get caught doing something and get suspended. On top of that, I have to face the facts; I was never good enough to win it. Those boys who get the Brownlow are true champions and out of my league. Mind you, winning medals wasn't why I played footy, for me it was about earning respect from the people I trained and played with.

As a young kid I loved everything about footy. Despite the competitiveness during the game, afterwards we would always have a hot dog and a can of Coke. We had an after-match function at 5 o'clock on Sunday night when the whole team would come together and our coach would announce the good players of the day. There was nothing better – the whole social aspect was fantastic. The lights would go on the oval and the kids would run around kicking goals, while the parents were getting pissed. This was a sense of community. I loved that close-knit feeling of having people around me who are all going for the same outcome, the same goal. That's why I still like being part of a team.

That said, we didn't have Auskick back then. It's a really fantastic organisation that do it really, really well. Nowadays, Auskick ensures the ball is given to every kid – they all get a kick. It's great. It's not all fun and games, though; it's a big-bucks business. I reckon the senior leagues should take a leaf out of the Auskick book as they'd probably get more success out of a team of 44 players if it was a little more fun and a lot less pressure. I know that is unrealistic, but at least the philosophy is right.

TAKING IT UP A NOTCH

As a junior player I only won a couple of best-and-fairest player trophies, but what made me stand out was when I was chosen to play Under-12s and Under-15s for Victoria, and then made the Under-15s All Australian Team. Under-12s for Victoria was a primary school competition where 1000 kids competed for 24 spots. They had a huge selection program. It involved going to Ivanhoe Grammar for training on a Sunday morning, which was about an hour's drive away. Mum took me every time, and we went backwards and forwards, playing games and training. This went on for quite some time. I made it into the team but didn't play all that well during the competition. I toured Albury-Wodonga in New South Wales to play all the different states. It was a big carnival. The other kids were a lot bigger than me and I played pretty averagely really, but I did the best I could. Just getting chosen was a coup. I was one of the 24 selected from all over Victoria, so that was pretty good.

Victorian selection made me a bit of a hero back in our local community with the story making it into the newspaper. That was my first back-page story and I was proud and excited that I had made the paper. When you are young you want to have your photo in the paper. Of course, it is a double-edged sword. At first you want to be recognised and get drafted, but then once that happens, it is sort of downhill from there when it comes to the press.

THE TAC CUP

In 1992, the junior football league in Victoria was revamped to what is now called the Victorian Schools Football League (VSFL) and the TAC Cup, which is where most of the drafted players are chosen. All the recruiters come and watch. I joined the TAC Cup competition when I was 14, and played for the Central Dragons. You can't choose your team; it all depends on your postcode and the zones. We had to drive 45 minutes to training, three times a week. My coach was an old chap called Slug Jordon – Ray Jordon – who is very well known in Melbourne. I was picked for his team but I was still a very young player so it was more of a training role that year. In saying that, once the finals came, I was put in a preliminary final to play on Aussie Jones, who was three years older than me, and a huge name back then because he was a certainty to be drafted to St Kilda.

We're talking about me playing in an Under-18 comp and I was 14, and still a small 60 kilograms – a jockey really. I played on Waverley Park, which at the time was St Kilda's home ground, but has been taken out of the AFL now. It was a special experience. I had sold *The Footy Record* there when I was 11 years old. Back then selling *The Footy Record* was a highly sought-after job for a young kid and to get it you had to do a normal paper round, which involved getting up at 4am and throwing papers six days a week. So each week I'd be at Waverley Park selling *Records* then go inside, put the pie rack on and sell pies. I used to watch Robert Harvey, Nathan Burke and Stewart Lowe while I was working, and years later ended up being their teammate when I played for St Kilda.

SO THE SACRIFICE BEGINS

I was attracted to these types of jobs at the footy club because I liked being around footy. Mind you, when the cricket season was on, I loved cricket more than footy. When I turned 14, I had a decision to make because I was a decent cricketer as well, having played for the district and state teams in cricket. I loved both sports, but when I did my law of averages, I worked out there were 12 players who played for Australia in cricket and there were 650 odd players who played AFL. So my chances to reach the top level were a lot better playing football. It wasn't a passionate decision, it was a simple calculation. I am that black and white in most areas, I don't have much grey at all. Once I made up my mind that was it. As a 14-year-old I saw football as a good career prospect.

Being serious about football meant making sacrifices from as early as the age of 10. I didn't know it at the time, but the sacrifice was massive, and there were no guarantees. Thousands of kids try to get drafted and only 90-odd kids are picked each year. I still wonder about the thousands who sacrificed themselves for those three or four years leading up to the draft and didn't get chosen. I gave up going out with my friends. If they went to a late session at the movies, I couldn't go as I had to get my sleep. I lost my social life altogether because my parents were so strict – they wanted me to succeed in footy. At this stage, the pressure was more parental than club-based.

That all changes, though, once you get involved with representative teams, such as the Victorian Under-15s or the All Australian Team. It especially changes when you join a TAC Cup team. Parents come under a huge amount of scrutiny from the club in relation to what their kids are doing. Clubs start telling parents what they should feed their children and when they should sleep; it's not subtle, parents actually meet with the coach and dietician. I started on a special diet when I was 14, which was necessary because the training regime was so high, I needed special food to give me the energy required.

It's not all sacrifice and doom and gloom. On the positive side, footy provided me with a good education about healthy living, as well as keeping me out of the party scene as I got older. In a sense it kept me off the streets; off the grog; and it also kept me away from smoking dope, the drug of choice of my friends when we were growing up. Our suburb was no worse than any others in Melbourne in the '90s, there were drugs everywhere just like there is today. I found living a healthy lifestyle just made me want to be healthier. Instead of having a pie with sauce after a game, I would replace that with a fresh roll or pasta, because I was learning that whatever I put in my mouth made a difference to how I performed.

As the umbrella organisation, the AFL runs all of the local competitions including the ones I played in. The purpose of the TAC Cup and the VSFL back then and still today, is to fast-track individual children as quickly as possible towards AFL football. Later on, when I was going through the VSFL Under-18 competition, about 30 per cent of those boys were getting drafted. That may have changed now, but it was pretty high back then. So the pressure became more

SO THE SACRIFICE BEGINS

intense the older we became to perform well on the football field and for parents to feed us well, to stop us going out and to keep us exercising. Even when I went away on Christmas holidays with my parents, I had to stick to a strict regime of training, and this was from 14 or 15 years of age.

It got to the stage where I was thinking I had to train on New Year's Eve to give myself an edge over my opponents. I remember one New Years Day, when I was 15 years old, doing a 10km run through the sand dunes of a Torquay back beach. Everyone else took those two days off. Mum and Dad were fully supportive of this because their view was always, the harder you worked the luckier you got. I trained like this for most of my AFL career knowing that a lot of the opposition players would not be doing this, so I was at least two training sessions up on them each year. A small thing, but mentally for me, it was huge.

At the time, I loved this life. I didn't resent it then but as time moved on I did start to resent the impact the sport was having on my life. Every footy player will have a different opinion on this, but I missed out in every aspect of my life other than footy. I never went to the 18th birthday party of any of my friends, not one. I never went to any because I was playing football and I was living in Western Australia. I missed all of my friends' 21st birthdays as well, I just used to send presents and cards. I missed that whole part of my youth while I just continued to play footy.

When I retired and separated from my wife I went off the deep end and part of it, I reckon, was because I wanted to be an 18-year-old again. The problem was, as a

29-year-old, people were pointing the finger saying *"you've lost the plot, you need help"*. Turns out they were right, but how little they knew about my life.

I wasn't asking anyone to feel sorry for me, because I certainly didn't feel sorry for myself, and I was doing what I loved at the time, but looking back it's remarkable to me – not one 18th birthday party, not one 21st party. Even my own 21st was put back six months because I was playing football and couldn't attend.

Imagine it.

CHAPTER 5
DREAMS COME TRUE

"Then it got to pick 12 which was the Fremantle Dockers. I had heard nothing from Fremantle, nothing, and then they called out my name... I think the first thing I did was put my face into my hands and think *"no way, Western Australia"*."

Getting an opportunity to play in a TAC Cup team at the age of 14 was incredible really. It's a real exception these days if they let a 15 or 16-year-old play because the intensity of the competition is similar to the Western Australian Football League (WAFL) Colts.

I had to leave the Central Dragons (now called Sandringham Dragons) after my zone changed and I went to a new team called the Oakleigh Chargers. Even though I wanted to stay with my original team, I had to make the change. It was disappointing because I'd played in a final with the Dragons and I'd been given an opportunity to play at the Under-18 level by Slug Jordon even though I was younger than everyone else. The only way I could have stayed was if

I'd had my mail sent to a different postcode. Really, though, it wasn't worth the risk. Football in Victoria is pretty serious stuff. Imagine a whole competition that's been running for 16/17 years purely to fast track junior footballers to play AFL footy and you get the idea.

So in 1995, when I was 15, I got rezoned to the Oakleigh Chargers. The coach was David Ackerley who played for the Sydney Swans in the VFL. David was a very hard taskmaster but because I had a reputation as an up-and-coming player, I expected to get a good go. David played me continuously in our first year and we got to play on the MCG in our first final. Although we lost the game, it was great to be playing on the hallowed turf.

I had previously been on the MCG as a 14-year-old in a Super Kick competition during half time of the Grand Final – I think Carlton and Essendon were playing. The aim was to kick the ball longest using your preferred foot and your non-preferred foot. There were 95,000 people watching and I won! I beat all these other guys from all over Victoria and won a shield and $2500 in prize money so I was pretty happy.

The second year with the Chargers was a very important year for me, it was 1996 and based on my performance of the previous year, I was looking to get drafted. The rules have changed now, and because I didn't turn 17 until late-May I would have had to wait another year. I understand this change was made to allow students to finish Year 12 and to limit the impact on them if they needed to move interstate.

Back then the school part didn't bother me as I had left school at the end of Year 11 to work with my step-Dad as an apprentice carpenter. I was getting up at 5 o'clock in the morning, working and then training three times a week, trying to get drafted as I worked hard unloading trucks and carting timber. I was so fatigued I found I really struggled that year, but as a young boy obsessed with footy nothing could slow me down and all I could think about was that every club was able to pick one 17-year-old on their list. So my chances of getting drafted were one in 16 that year.

I knew that if I wasn't successful as a 17-year-old I would hopefully get drafted the following year because this is the prime two-year window you really have to get in. So what happened in this crucial first year? I played very averagely. I played in the back pocket, which was a position I wasn't used to at that stage of my career. When you are trying to be selected, you need to shine; you need to run; you need to kick goals and that back pocket position didn't allow me to do all of those things.

Luckily for me the rules then changed for the TEAL Cup, which is the AFL National Under-18 championships, and it included Under-17s, so I was eligible for TEAL Cup selection. Even though I was having an ordinary year my reputation meant they kept me on until the last cut. It got down to the last two boys to represent Victoria metropolitan, and I only just scraped through to get into the squad. I was the 22nd player picked, which was not good but I had made it. During the TEAL Cup I was able to reverse form and play on the wing, which was my favoured position. We won the competition, and for me it was a fairytale ending. We played in the grand final against South Australia on the MCG and, with three seconds to go in the match, I got the ball on the 50m mark and banged it through for a goal. The siren went, we'd won the grand final and I had the last kick scoring my third goal.

That kick got me drafted, there is no doubt about it, and it still gets played on TV today. On the day I had a real battle playing on Stuart Dew who went on to have a fantastic career playing for Port Adelaide and Hawthorn. He kicked two goals and I kicked three, it was a real old-fashioned tussle. I will never forget it. It was a great feeling to know what I had achieved when I was very much under the pump to perform.

From there, I was chosen for the All-Australian Team, which meant an automatic invitation to the Draft camp. It's a two-day camp where you go to seminars and they put you through a fitness regime like no other. Of course, at that age, I had no idea about my anxiety or struggles with dealing with new people. What I did know is that I was extremely nervous and my way of handling this was to act like the class clown.

The Draft camp is run by the AFL and it felt a little bit like we were cattle. Recruiting officers and coaches from every team attend the camp to evaluate everyone. We were put through a psychiatric test, which I probably failed, and had to meet the psychologist from each club. It's at this time when players are pinpointed by certain clubs. Thinking back, Fremantle didn't even speak to me at the Draft camp but coaches, recruiting officers and psychologists from several other clubs all sat down and had a chat with me.

At that stage, I still hadn't given much thought to who I wanted to play for. I think every young player acknowledges that once you sign the Draft papers you are signing on to go anywhere in Australia. You don't have any say in it. My preference would have been to stay in Melbourne because I am from a pretty tight family and I was only 17 years old. I was a passionate Essendon supporter at the time, so Essendon would have been a fairytale. It all works out for a reason and, when I look back, going to Fremantle gave me an opportunity to play at the top level very early in my career. In all honesty, though, I got played well ahead of time and the club should have spent more time working me up to that level of footy.

But getting back to the Draft camp, we had to jump through all sorts of hoops; things like strength testing, vertical jumps to show how high you can go and a lot more. People were constantly watching and it was all recorded, which was pretty intimidating. Back then I was a skinny whippet, so not very strong (I bench-pressed 75kg, compared to 135kg when I was in the AFL). During the agility tests we were timed going through cones; then they put us into a dark room for reflex testing. We had to tap the lights on a board to demonstrate our reaction time. I enjoyed this, it was a bit of fun, but the anxiety crept in during an endurance test. My answer to these nerves was to talk incessantly and play down the importance of the tests to everyone.

BLACK

Imagine a bunch of 17 year old boys waiting to start the test, and there is good old Heath bagging the whole thing and saying he didn't really give a shit about the outcome. It turned out to be an old-fashioned beep test where you run 20m and the beeps get quicker. I ended up doing quite well. I ran a 14/10, which would have put me among the top 10. My behaviour then was as much about intimidating the other players, which became common practice for me during my AFL years, but that natural drive to downplay things still kicks in when I get nervous. Maybe it's about not setting the bar too high for myself and in the eyes of those around me, so if I do fail, I can say, *"I told you I'd fuck it up"*.

Reputation was a big part of the drafting process as well. Reputation based mainly on your skill and playing ability is everything in footy when you are young. This is why all the games I played in my teens were so important. What the people at the Draft saw in me from the start, apart from being fast, were my kicking skills and the ability to win the ball on the ground because I was small and always a good tackler. I'm left-handed, so I'm a left-foot kicker, which is a bit different and meant I could set-up the play and hit the forward on the chest. So testing aside, the camp was spent training and playing footy and being watched – the whole time.

Many of our results were announced during the camp, so we knew roughly how we were going. Recently drafted AFL players came in and talked to the group and I would do the same thing two years after I was selected. There were seminars and talks on diet and drugs and alcohol. We even had media training. Sandy Roberts, who still works for Channel 7, interviewed every single player and took us through the interviewing process so we had some experience of what it was like to be interviewed by a professional media person. The cameras were there, everything was there - it was great but very full on. Strangely enough, talking to the media did not bother me or bring on any anxiety attacks, I saved that for the footy field.

I was hopeful that I'd get an opportunity to play on an AFL list either that year or the next. You do have some idea because you get an amazing amount of feedback from the people who talk to you. You also get letters sent to your house from the different clubs to let you know whether they are interested in you. Despite all of that, it still doesn't mean you are over the line. I received letters from about 10 different clubs but it didn't mean anything because none of them ended up picking me. A lot of the kids get their hopes up but because there is never any formal commitment at that stage, their hopes get smashed fairly quickly. I remember talking to the recruiting guys from the Sydney Swans, Geelong and the Western Bulldogs the day before the Draft and all of them said *"when our pick comes we are going to select you tomorrow"*.

Of course, the Draft all depends on where a team finishes on the ladder the previous year. The bottom club gets first pick, the second bottom club gets second pick and so on. This makes the competition fairer but it is tough if you are the best player and you go to the worst club. To make things even more complicated, there is trade week, which is seven days where established players from each team get traded.

When it comes to the established players, contracts mean nothing. When the club agrees to trade you, the negotiations start and in some cases the receiving club has to take over the payments on the contract. Salary caps also come into the equation. Let's just say for example, you might be released to go to Fremantle but if you were on say $400,000 at St Kilda and Fremantle can only pay $350,000 because they are limited by the cap, you can still leave St Kilda, be paid the $350,000 by Fremantle, but St Kilda have to pay the $50,000.

When I played there were many players who were playing for one club, but still getting paid by their previous employer. It is all about list management. Each team has a list manager and at the end of the year they will look at the amount of game experience and/or the age of players in the team and if a lot are over 30 years, they just wean down. You need a full-time list manager to keep the list useful enough to ensure that you don't drop to the bottom of the ladder.

So trade week and the Draft go hand in hand. For me, there were whispers and innuendo about the team I might have played for. It actually became really hard to keep my head above water. Back then the Draft was shown on TV, so I had to sit in my lounge room and just wait to see if my name was called. In those days that was how you found out if you had been chosen. Foxtel rang me just before the Draft and asked if they could come to my house and film my response. Although it's happened several times since then, I

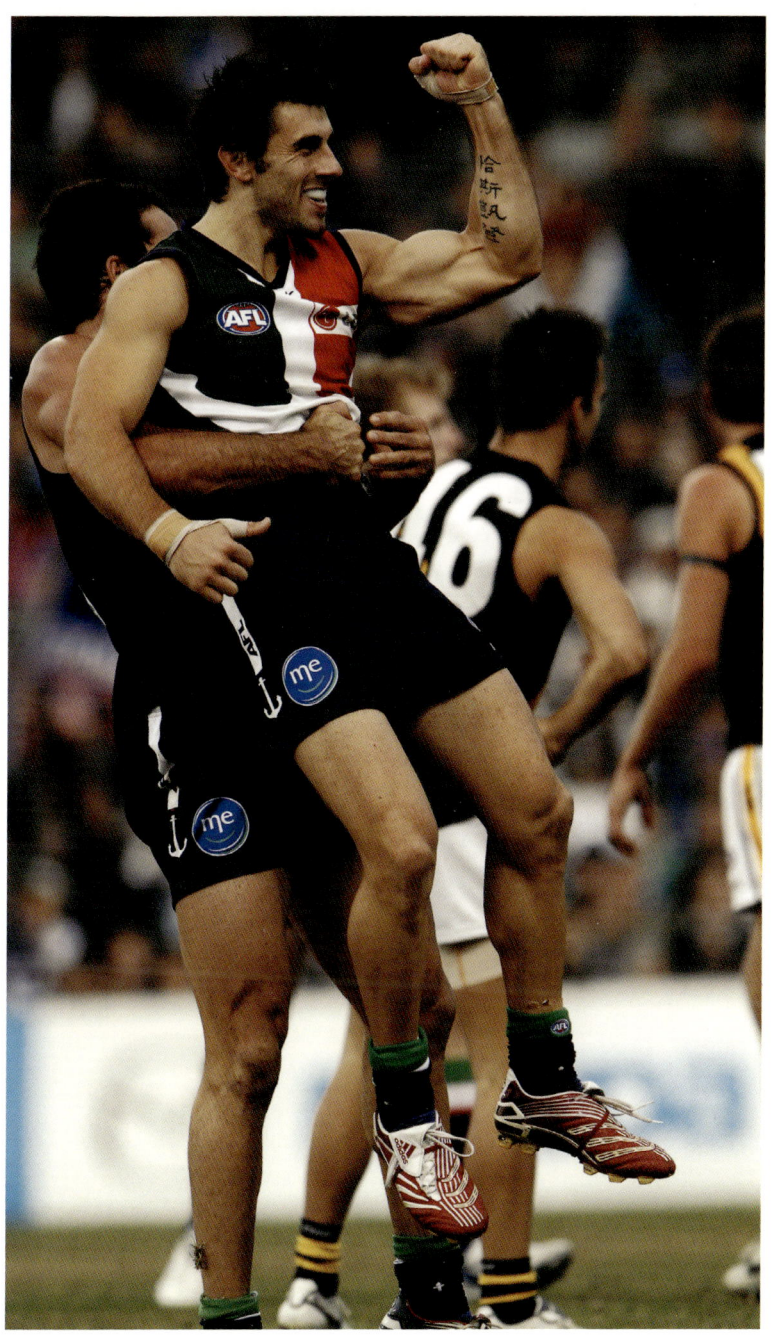

This was taken just after I kicked a goal against Richmond at Subiaco Oval in 2007. I am being lifted by my mate, Dean Solomon (Solly). NEWSPIX/JODY D'ARCY

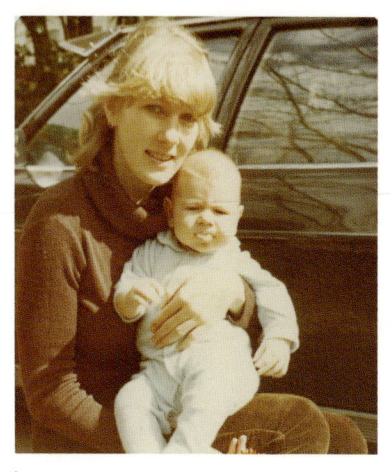

Mum and me at Nan and Pop Eastwood's house, Ashburton, Victoria, 1979.

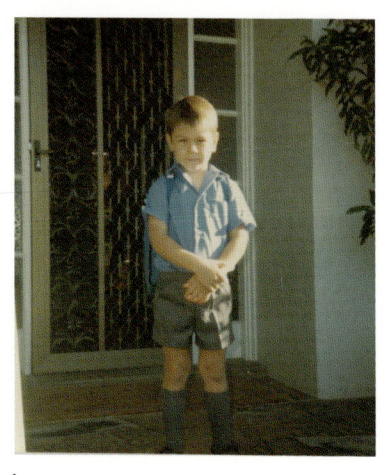

On my first day of school, aged 5 in 1984.

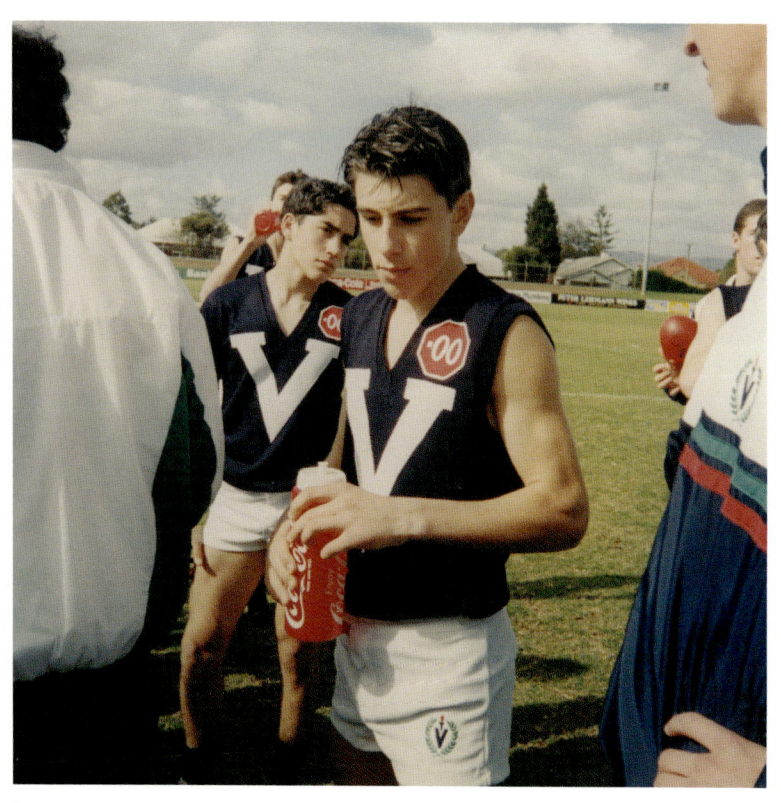

The start of the footy dream - playing for Victoria "The Big V" in the Under-15 side in 1994.

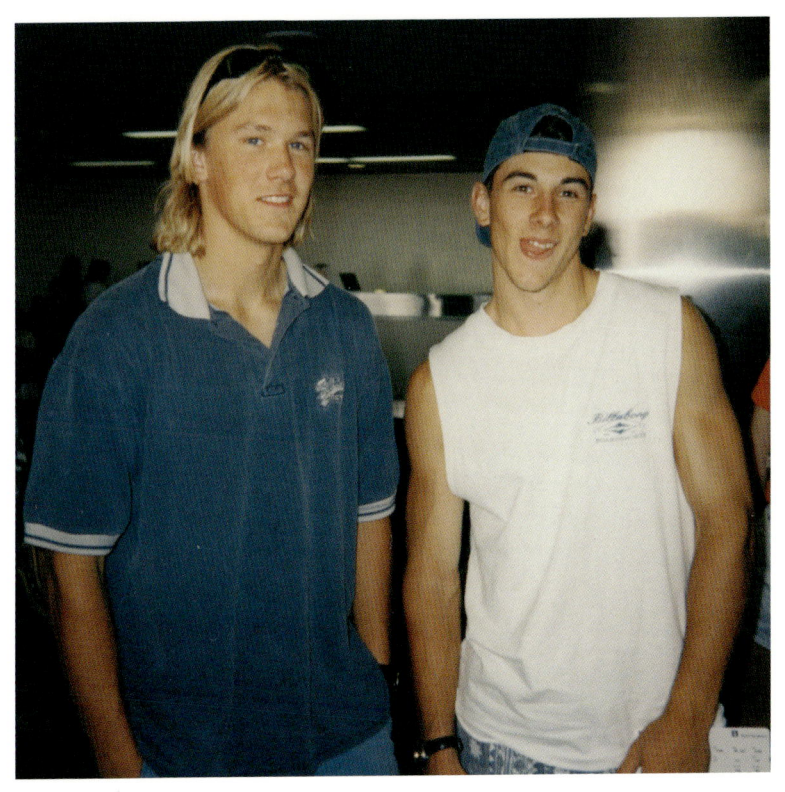

With Jess Sinclair at the Melbourne airport on our first trip to Perth after being drafted for Fremantle in 1996.

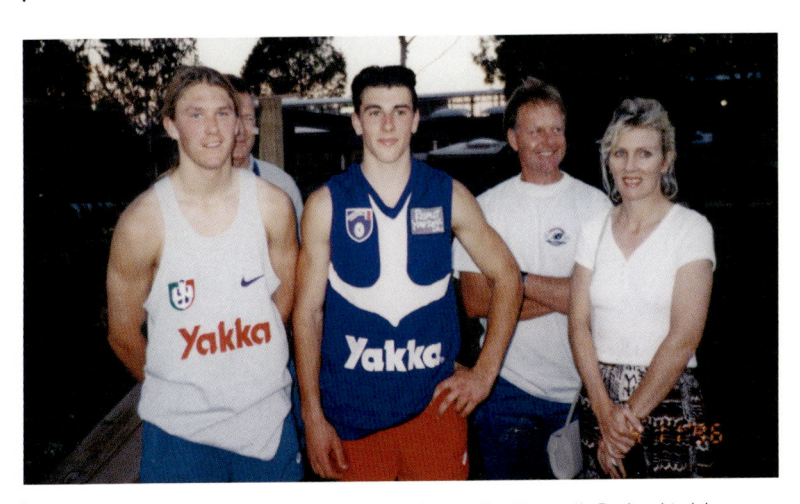

Jess Sinclair and I with my step-Dad and Mum after our first Fremantle Dockers' training session in 1996.

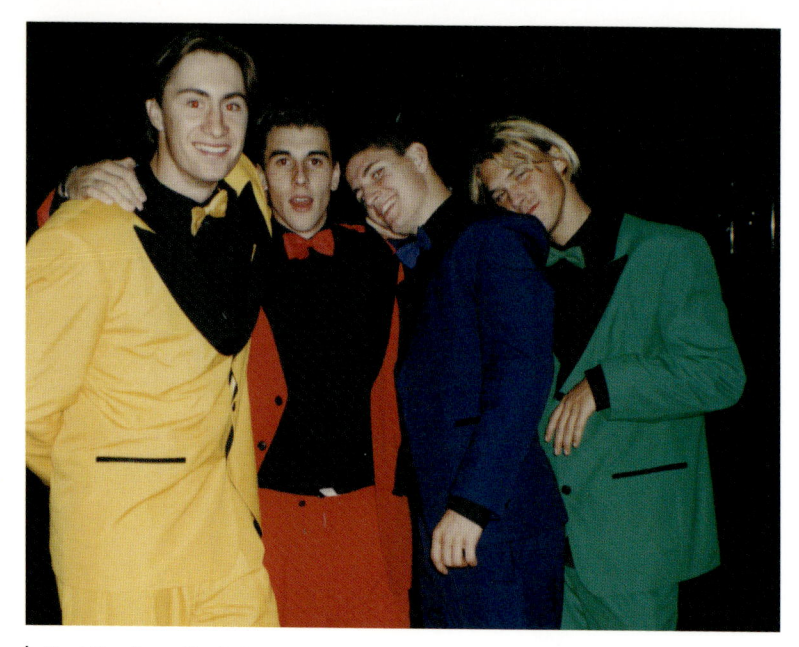

Trent Carroll, me, Brodie Holland and Jess Sinclair got ourselves into a bit of trouble for dressing like The Wiggles at a Fremantle Football Club Black Tie function in 1998.

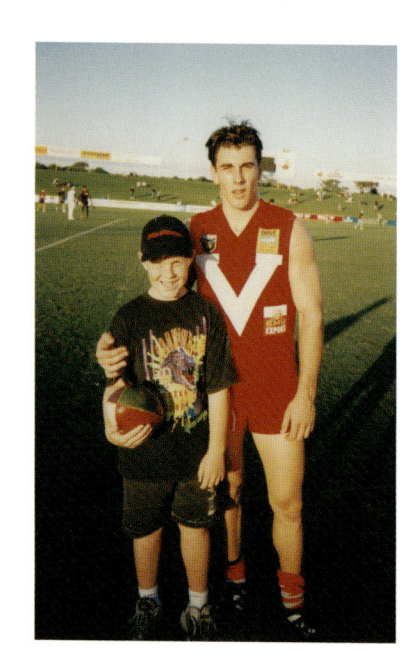

With my younger brother Dean in Perth, 1999. I was returning from injury, so I played for South Fremantle in the WAFL.

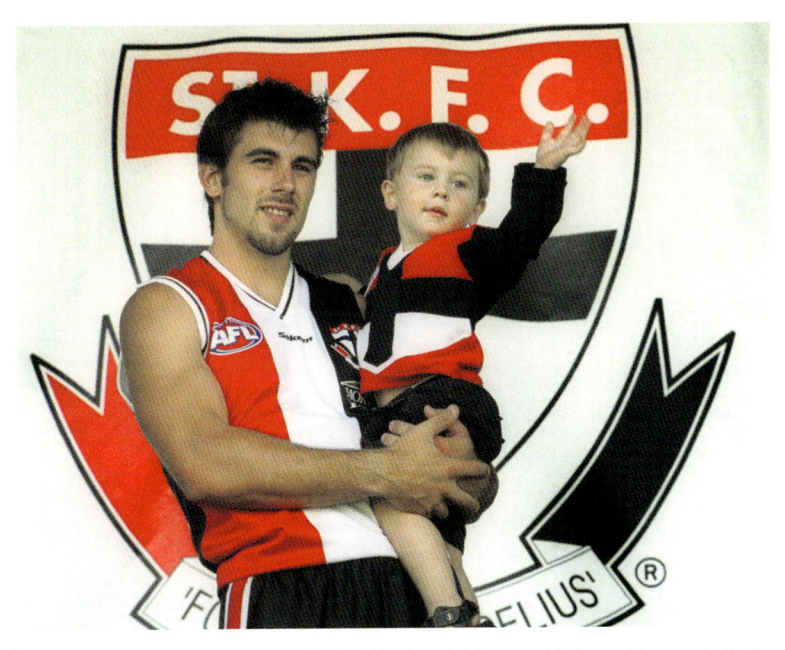

This was taken at a St Kilda family day in 2003. I am holding my eldest son, Chayce, who had done a poo in his nappy which was running down my arm. NEWSPIX/KAREN DODD

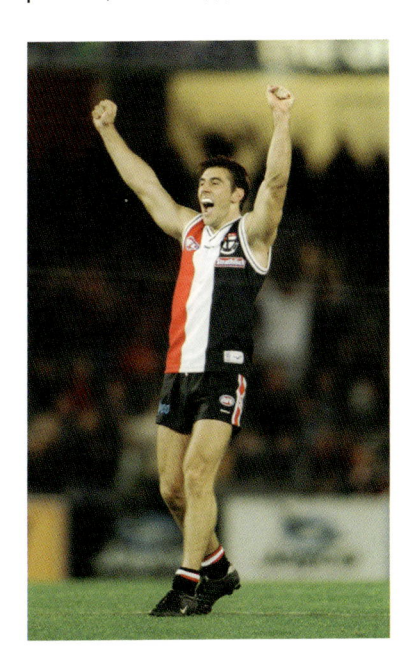

I was pretty happy about kicking a goal against Carlton in my first game for St Kilda, Round 1 of 2002. We won this game 89 to 65. NEWSPIX/NEWS LIMITED

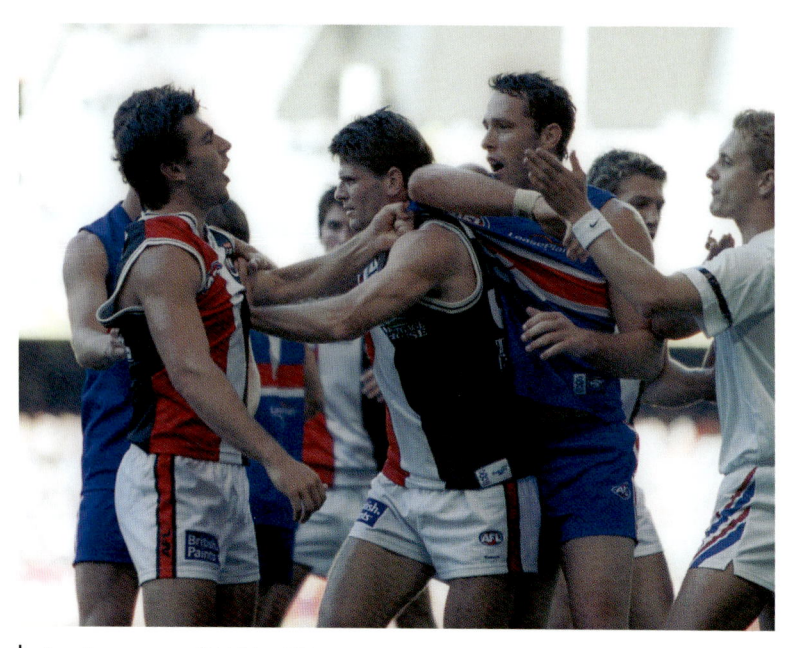

One of my many on-field fights. This one was during the first quarter break against Western Bulldogs in 2003. Seconds before this photo, I received a right hook from Ryan Hargreaves which left me with a hairline fracture in my jaw. NEWSPIX/GEORGE SAL

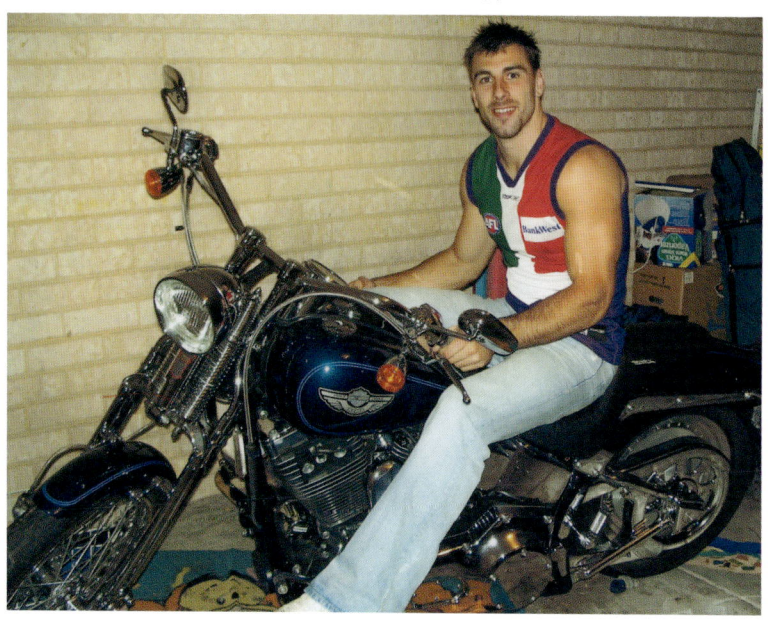

Sitting on my much-loved Harley Davidson at home in Perth 2007.

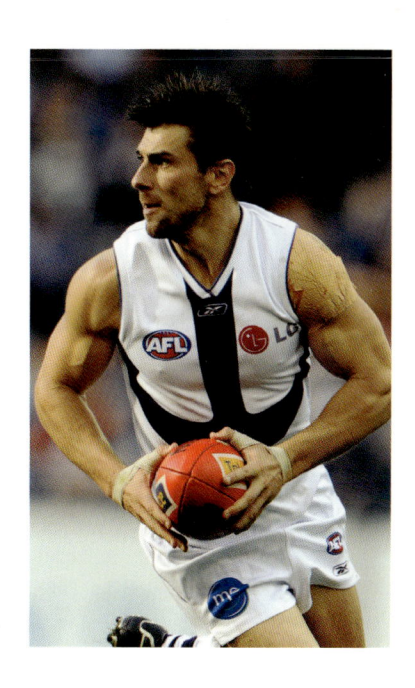

Playing for Fremantle in 2008. I retired in August of the same year.
NEWSPIX/STEPHEN HARMAN

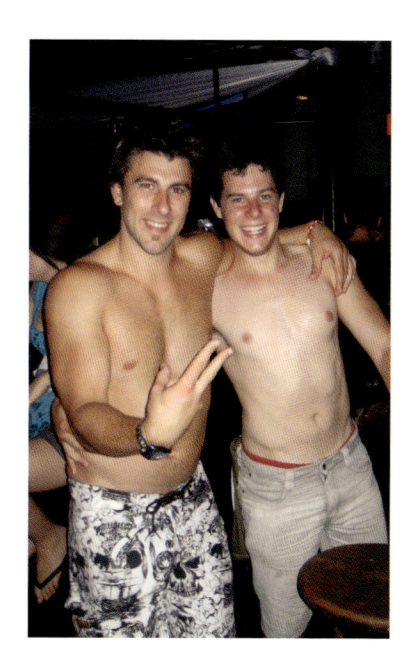

A night I would rather forget with my brother Shaun in Bali, January 2009. This was taken several hours before my huge fight with the Russians.

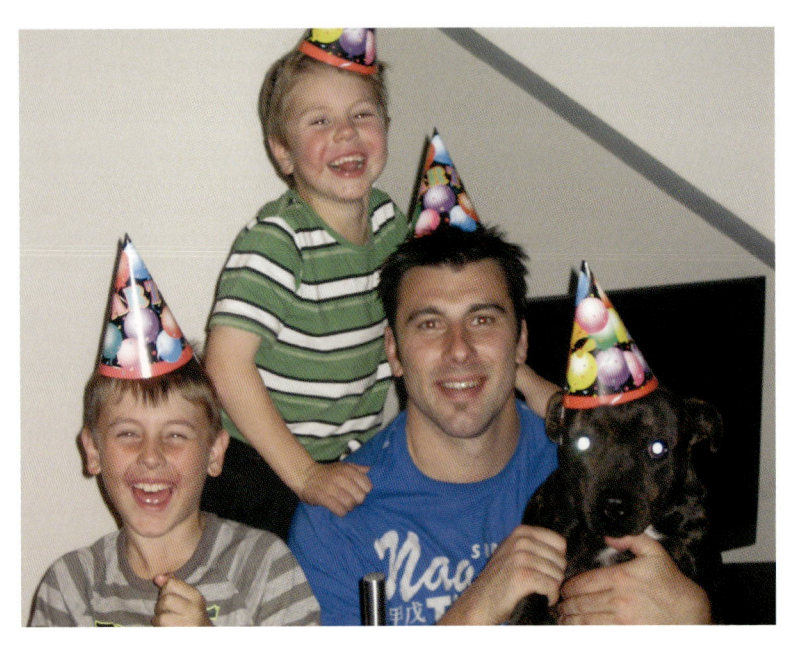

Celebrating my 30th birthday with Chayce, Cayden and my dog Sarge, in May 2009. Sarge was killed later that year.

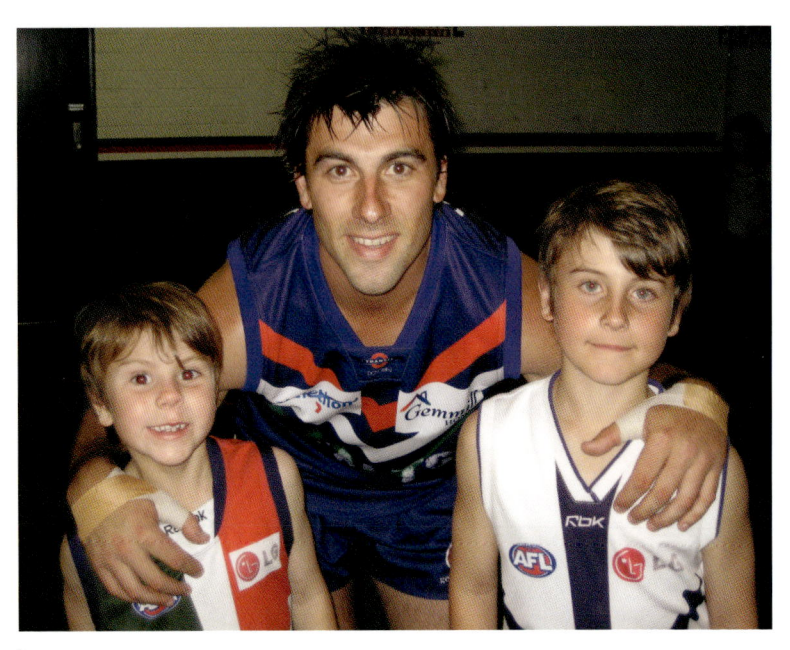

With my boys, Cayden and Chayce at the 2010 West Coast "OWLS" vs Fremantle "Old Salts", a game played in honour of former West Coast Eagle, Chris "Mainy" Mainwaring.

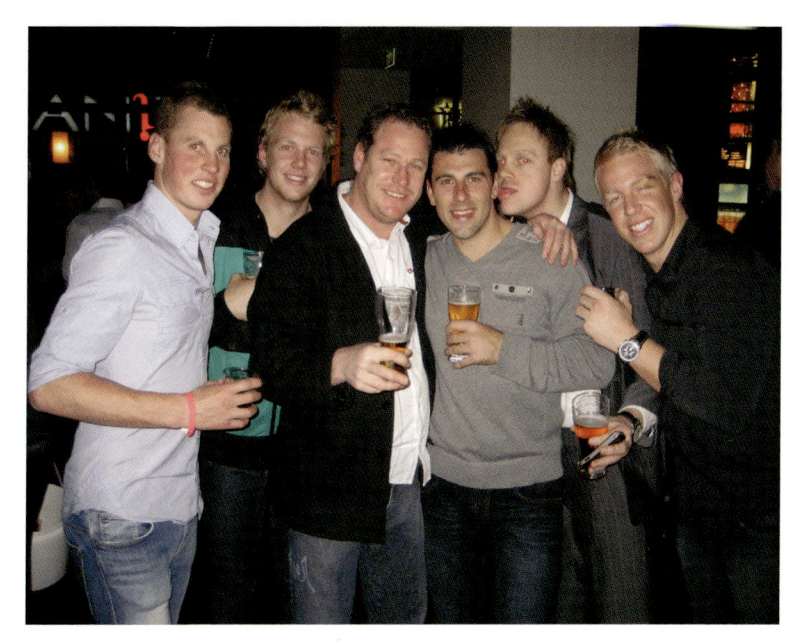

At the Melbourne Casino after the 2010 EJ Whitten Legends Game with Weeksy, Jace, Sully, Paul Nelson and Dean.

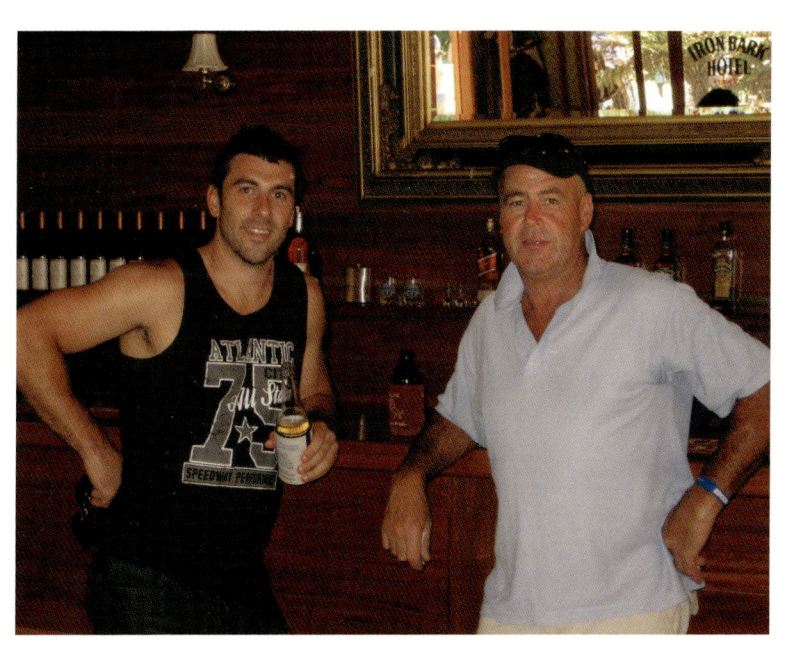

Me and Dad relaxing on a bar in 2011 – something we've always done well.

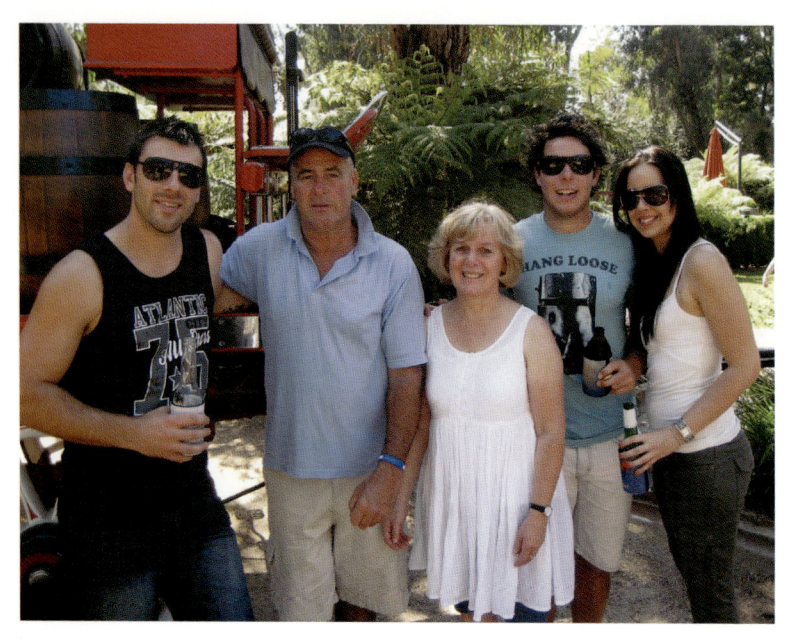

Out in the bush with Dad, my step-Mum Jan, brother Shaun and his girlfriend Peta. This was taken in 2011.

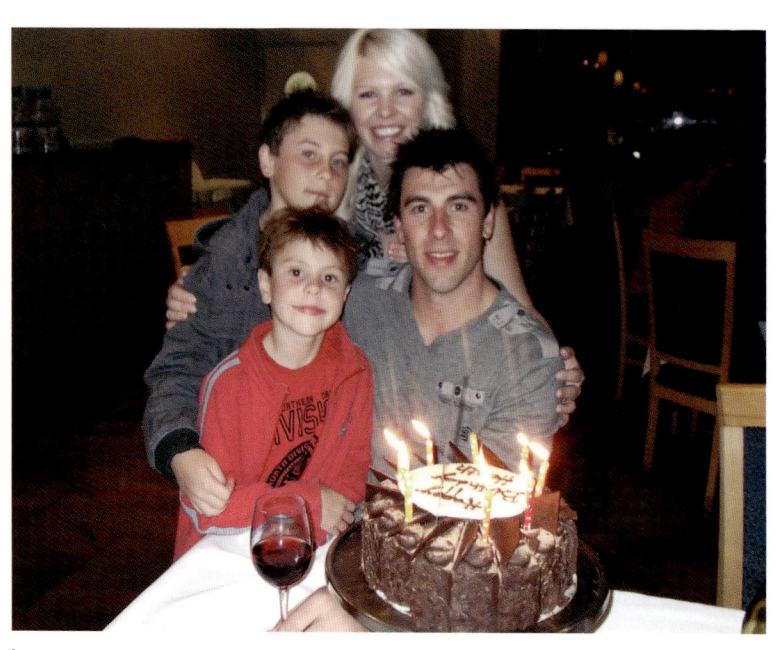

Surrounded by the ones I love the most – with Asha, Chayce and Cayden in Australind, 2011.

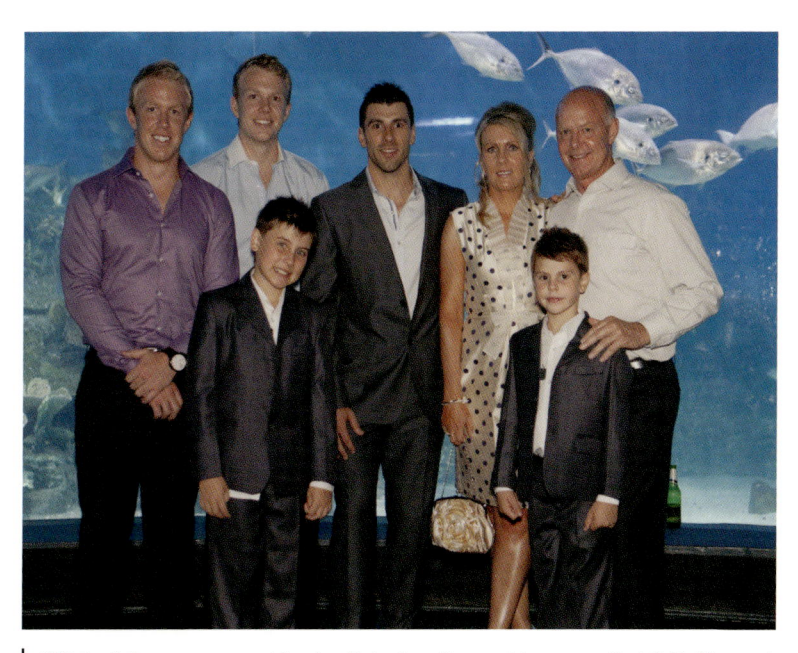

With the Kelly gang on my wedding day. My brothers Dean and Jace are on the left. My Mum and step-Dad are on the right. My sons, Chayce and Cayden are the two handsome ones in the front.
COURTESY OF THE BANK STUDIO

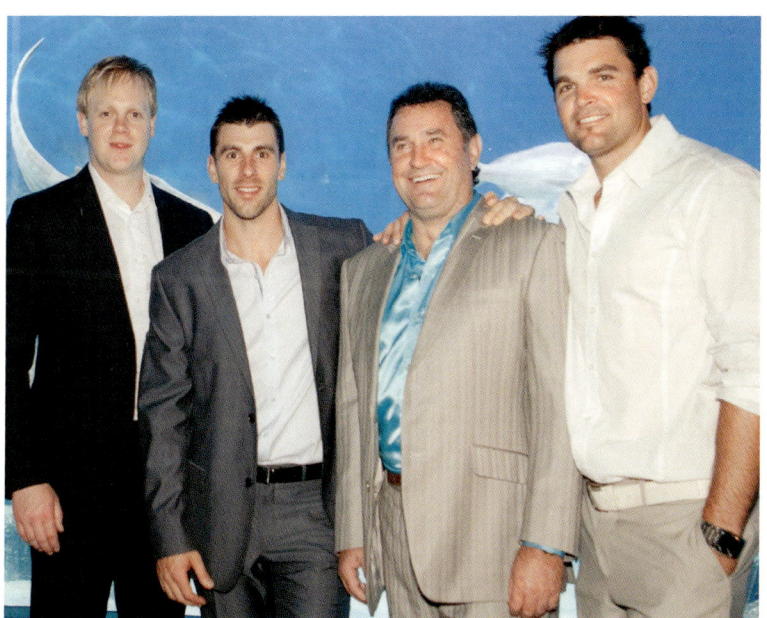

With my mates on New Year's Eve. Paul Nelson is on the left, John Rankin (JR) and his son Chad are on the right. COURTESY OF THE BANK STUDIO

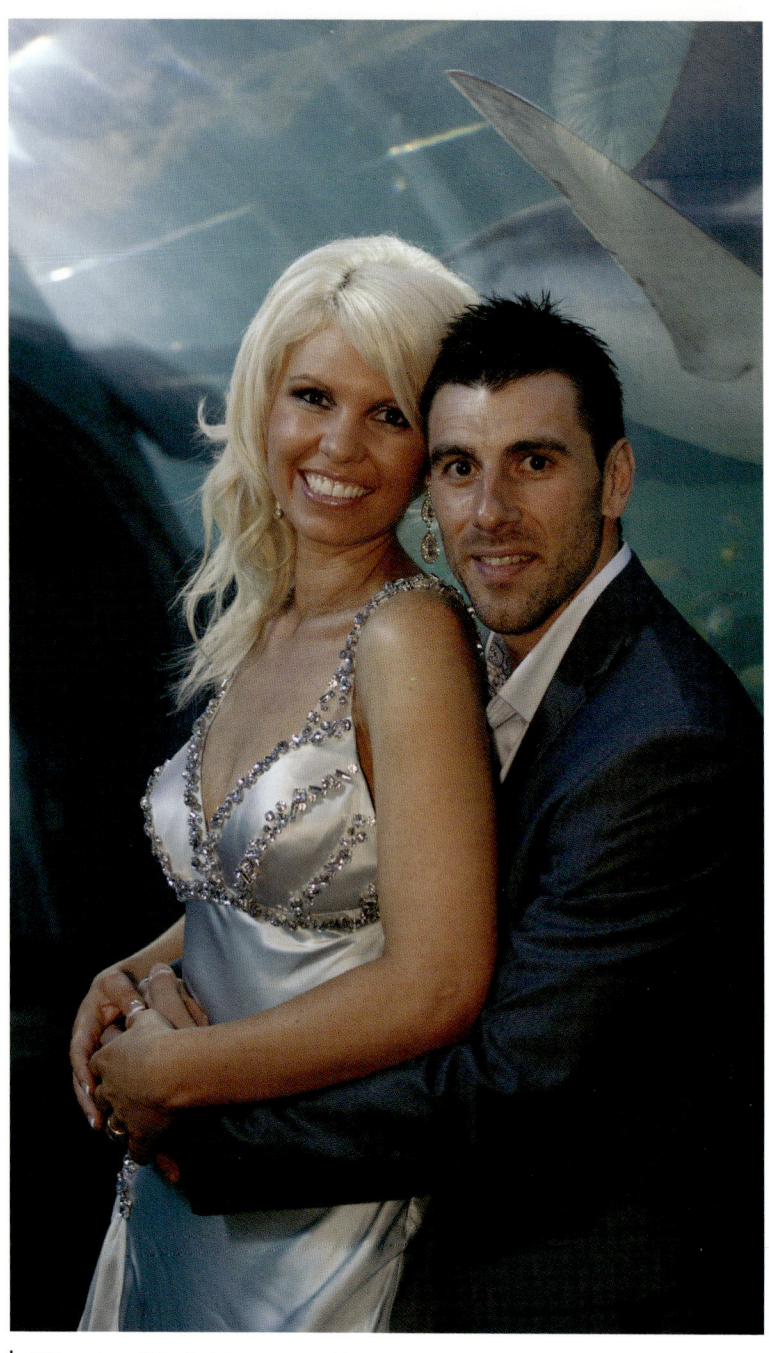

With my beautiful wife Asha on our wedding day at the Melbourne Aquarium, New Year's Eve 2011. COURTESY OF THE BANK STUDIO think I was probably one of the first players to do this. I've seen times when Foxtel has been at a player's house and the poor kid didn't get drafted. It is not a guarantee but, back then, I just thought I was the duck's nuts.

On the day of the Draft my whole family came over to my parents' house. I was there in my work clothes because that is what Foxtel wanted. Claire, my girlfriend at the time, was next to me and there was family galore all over the place – 30-plus people were all on the gas, partying. I remember sitting there, extremely nervous, watching it on TV. I sat there for 10 picks and the next one up was the Western Bulldogs, who only the night before had promised to pick me. Bang, they didn't call out my name. Then it got to pick 12, which was the Fremantle Dockers. I had heard nothing from Fremantle, nothing, and then they called out my name. I was already very tense and coming from a family that is so tight, the first thing I did was put my face into my hands and I just sat there; I was like *"no way, Western Australia"*.

My family was bawling, Claire was sobbing, everyone was like *"oh no, shit no"*. That lasted for about a minute, with me in the middle of it all on my own. It was totally out of control. I think everyone then thought *"oh shit, the camera is here"*, so then it turned into *"oh wow, that's great"* and they all gave me a hug. I have the footage of this, it is a classic moment, and I am young, only 17, it is horrible really. Then it kicked in that I was drafted and the dream had come true.

It was such a confusing time. I felt terrible on one hand because my life had just been tipped upside down. I was really involved with Claire and I knew that it was not going to work long-distance. Obviously it meant moving to Western Australia and doing a lot more flying, and I had a serious fear of flying. All I could think was *"fuck, I've got to fly, how am I going to do this?"*. I also felt let down by Fremantle because there had been no contact at all, absolutely no word, I didn't even know the team song.

But before I knew it, their recruiting officer Phil Smart and the general manager Gerard McNeal had made the trek out to my home in Mulgrave to introduce themselves. I let them in and there they calmly sat in the lounge room surrounded by people who wanted to rip their heads off. It's weird really, both parties not wanting to let their guard down and these two guys were very much trying to create this impression of Fremantle being a total winner's club and wasn't I lucky to be chosen by them?

So Freo had chosen two of us local boys – me and my friend Jess Sinclair - and they also selected a West Aussie, Matthew Clukus. In that year there were about 90 draft picks and I was number 12, and on top of that I was Fremantle's number one draft pick so that was a good result. That said, I doubt I was at the top of Fremantle's list, there were better players than me in the Draft. But anyway, after I had put my doubts aside, we all started to celebrate and everyone was pretty happy. Towards the end of Draft night, and after the Dockers people had left to go see Jess and tell him the good news, I went out with my friends to a mate's dad's pub with all of us wearing the Freo scarves and other paraphernalia from Phil.

DREAMS COME TRUE

Don't ask me what happened that night; when I woke up in the morning I had no idea of what had gone on. But even though things were foggy, I did know one thing, I had my chance at last to live the dream – to play AFL footy.

CHAPTER 6
WELCOME TO THE AFL

"It ended up being the only senior grand final I have ever played in and won. It was in my first year of footy. Can you believe it? It was a fairytale, but the next year in 1998, I was struck down by injury and only played one match. They call them the 'Footy Gods' and they are up there somewhere, they'll take it away from you as quick as they gave it to you."

The Draft was in November 1996 and within two weeks, Jess Sinclair and I were in Fremantle. We came over with our families and got shown around Perth, checked out the Dockers' training facilities and got to meet the team. I had never been to Perth so everything was new.

I loved Fremantle as soon as I saw it. If I'm going to be upfront, the first things to make a real impression on me were all the pubs. The cafe strip was still buzzing and freshly painted from the America's Cup. As Jess and I were new recruits from Victoria we were automatically held in high regard from Fremantle fans and the media. As soon as we got off the plane there were television cameras everywhere. We were a pretty big thing, everyone wanted to know what the Victorians were like. You have to remember, back then the Dockers had only been going for two years and, as with West Coast, most of the line-up was West Aussie boys. I was interviewed straight away by the papers and TV, the whole shebang, so it was pretty full-on right from the word go. I was on the back page of *The West Australian* newspaper the next day with *"This is our new recruit"* – pretty daunting stuff for a 17-year-old.

I never grew up near the ocean, so the whole beach culture was new to me. When we first arrived we ended up living in Scarborough after we were billeted with Theresa Burton, Matthew Burton's mum. Matthew, better known as Spider Burton, played for Fremantle and was the tallest player in the AFL at the time. Jess was 18 and I was 17 and we both stayed at Theresa's house, which was a fair way from Fremantle where a lot of the other team members lived. It was made all the harder as neither Jess nor I had our driver's licence. In Victoria you had to be 18 to get your licence, which is different to Western Australia where you could get it at 17. One of the first things that happened was we got taken by a copper, a Dockers' supporter of course, and an excellent bloke who has since passed away, to a country town to do our test. Out of respect for those no longer with us, I can't give too much detail, but let's just say the process wasn't too rigorous, and before we knew it we had our licences.

Obviously the most intimidating thing for me on that first trip was to meet the team. Ben Allen was the captain of the Dockers at the time. He was an older player, who had been a champion at Hawthorn, and I ended up rooming with him a lot on the away games. I got on well with Ben and would pick his brains when we travelled. I asked him so many questions and he would always take the time to answer them for me.

He was a fairly intense person who just led from the front on the field. Although I probably didn't appreciate it at the time, Ben had reached the end of his playing career because his body was starting to let him down. Before the matches in his last year, he'd have the physio machine working over his knee and it was quite sad to see such a strong, brilliant legend of the game compromised and brought down that way. I mean he was only 29 years old, still fantastic on the field, yet it was all coming to an end. It was an eye opener for a young 17-year-old just starting his career. Funnily enough, my body also played a part, at about a similar age, in bringing my career to an end. Ben's still in footy, of course, he's now on the Board at the Fremantle Dockers.

Another well known name in Perth is Gerard Neesham, who was the coach at the time I joined. He gave me the opportunity to play extremely early and I was quite intimidated by him, mainly because he was my first AFL coach and you just don't know shit when you are young and that makes it scary. Another peculiarity about Gerard was that he incorporated house building into our training regime. Many of us ended up lugging bricks and other building materials around his Bicton home. It's probably safe to say that if anything ever went wrong with his house in the future, he could fairly blame the Fremantle Dockers and their building skills, or lack thereof.

Although I was initially intimidated by Gerard, the players were supportive and welcoming, but starting up was still one of the most daunting things I'd ever experienced. Nothing can prepare you for it. It was still old-school footy, so at that time of the year training hadn't yet started, so I only met a few players initially. Ben took Jess and I and our parents to a restaurant where we were made to feel like superstars. I thought I was the king of the world. That is the way they do it initially but little did I know that when I got into it I was just one of the many. It was all about making me feel welcome and reassuring my parents that I was going to be all right in a new city so far from home. So I went back to Victoria with my parents and I had another two weeks to get my shit together before I returned to Western Australia for good.

From day one at the club, it was full on. The first day of training, Jess and I had a 4km time trial with the rest of the team. We hadn't met many players at that stage, but I ran my guts out and ended up doing really well. My good performance in the run was in some part down to fear and anxiety – I was that scared. Even during this training there were die-hard fans watching us, which was all new to me. Beryl and Stuart Hogan – two very loyal Dockers' supporters – introduced themselves to me and my family and asked me for my autograph, which was a shock because it was the first time it had ever happened. Beryl told me I would be famous, which was very embarrassing but at the same time also encouraging. This euphoria associated with fans quickly wore off, mind you.

I think one of the most intimidating things on that first day was that most of the players were men and we were still just boys. That's one thing the WAFL has over the Victorian set-up, it's at a higher level and played with more intensity than the Under-17s in Victoria. On top of that, some of the guys at the club had already had significant AFL careers. Guys like Ben Allen, Stephen O'Reilly and Peter Mann were great players who had come back to Fremantle from other AFL clubs.

Initially I was aligned to South Fremantle, so the first few weeks of my career in the West, I played for Souths. All pre-season, which is three months or more, I trained with the Freo boys. Once Round 1 came, I trained with the Dockers on Monday, Tuesday and Wednesday and obviously I didn't make the team for the first game, so on Thursday I trained with South Fremantle, and had to meet all the players on that team. Again, I didn't know anyone, but the South Fremantle guys were great, and although there were a couple of young guys I was one of the youngest players in a predominantly older team.

In my first WAFL game, we travelled south to play the new team in the competition, Peel Thunder, for their first ever game in 1997. We went to Rushton Park, in Mandurah, and ended up winning by 138 points. With five minutes to the final siren, I got reported for striking, but I got off the charge. I was getting roughed up by my opponent so I punched him in the head. I went to the Tribunal, and there was video evidence, but even though they found me guilty they only reprimanded me. I didn't understand that at the time and I still don't. I got a good dressing-down by the Dockers though, considering we were 138 points up. I think what happened was that I expected to play better and I felt frustrated. That was my first experience of WAFL – getting reported in my first match and playing at Mandurah in front of a huge crowd. It absolutely lived up to my expectations.

The following Monday morning I had to sit down with our recruiting officer, who had taken it upon himself to be a father figure to Jess and I. We dissected the whole game at length and he berated me for losing my cool in the last five minutes. I knew I had done the wrong thing but it felt like a double blow. That said, it is the culture of the AFL to criticise before praising, and they pick the players they know can take it. I took it squarely on the chin and the fact is it made me play better and smarter the next time. The 'coach culture' will never change and it's really up to the psychologists to pick up the pieces later on.

PLAYING WITH THE BIG BOYS

By Round 4, Gerard Neesham picked me for the Dockers' team and, bang, I was in the AFL. I was still only 17 years old – a month away from my 18th birthday.

Looking back, I played my first AFL game pretty prematurely. With the way Fremantle was going at the time and with the list we had, I was probably given the opportunity to play AFL more quickly than many of my mates who had been drafted to the Melbourne AFL clubs.

Ideally, if the list is healthy, you should have nearly a year at WAFL level to get used to the bigger bodies.

Up until 2006, we were always the little brother down the road from West Coast. West Coast were the dominant team – they had more members and more success. In more recent years, Fremantle has started to win Derbies. Freo has been able to control and intimidate West Coast on the field; it has attracted as many members and financially it is going well. We've caught up on all levels except finals and winning premierships and, let's face it, ultimately that is what it is all about.

Initially, coming from Melbourne, I didn't get caught up in the 'Local Derby' and the whole scene which surrounded it. I tell you what, though, it doesn't take long to get consumed by Derby week and what it means to WA people. I think it only took me about six months to realise that there was a real rivalry between West Coast and Fremantle, and north and south of the river.

Back then, when the Dockers were new, it was pretty damn scary playing on the field during a Derby. We were a skinny, slight, young team and West Coast had John Worsfold, Chris Waterman and Peter Matera – they were huge. We looked like little boys and they looked like men. They just intimidated us. In my first Dockers versus West Coast practise match at South Fremantle Oval in 1997, I came up against Guy McKenna. All I remember was warming up at the other end of the ground, shitting myself that Guy was about 20kg heavier than me and at any opportunity I was sure he would try and intimidate me. In his defence, I don't think he was unnecessarily brutal, but when it came to the crunch, if those guys wanted to win the footy, I couldn't stop them.

There was no love-loss between the players from the two Perth AFL teams then and even now. They know where we hang out and we know where they hang out and there is not much social stuff between the teams. I think come finals time, the mentality of west versus east comes in. If Fremantle's out maybe a few of the boys might go for West Coast. I definitely don't, I would go for a Victorian team.

In those early years, when we used to get smashed by West Coast, I was fortunate to be involved in the first ever Dockers' win against West Coast in Round 16, 1999. It was huge. In the lead-up to the game, the team still had massive doubts that we could beat West Coast. But on that day it came down to two major factors – one, Anthony Modra, and two, the weather. It was a wet day and it brought West Coast down to our level.

After that night we were treated like Hollywood stars. We arrived at our local pub, The Left Bank, and there were TV cameras and flashing cameras and people everywhere. We walked straight up to the top deck and were treated like superstars. It was stupid really because even though we won the Derby, the Eagles ended up playing in the semi-finals while we missed out. But looking back it was fantastic, I'll never forget it. After The Left Bank we went to Zanzibar (a Fremantle nightclub) and although the bar was shut, they let the team in, and we got stuck into celebrating the win. Everyone was so proud of us.

WELCOME TO THE AFL

The next most memorable Derby was what infamously came to be known as the Demolition Derby of 2000. It is well documented that Clive Waterhouse had leaked to the press before bounce down that *"blood would be spilt"*, which set the whole tone for the game. Enough has been said about that game in various forums, but for history's sake, let's just say I felt comfortable in playing a hard game, which involved a physical presence on the field. The end result really said it all, seven of us were fined for being involved in a melee, and I copped the maximum $4000 fine. I'm happy to say we won the game by a point.

But getting back to my first game with the Dockers, which was against Richmond. It was the first game I played in front of my family at Princes Park, which is Carlton's home ground although they don't play AFL there anymore. Richmond weren't that flash at the time, so I think we only just went down to them. I actually played on a guy called Chris Bond who left Richmond and later would be captain of Fremantle. He was my first AFL opponent and I was playing on the wing. Jess Sinclair made his debut in Round 10, I think, so I was ahead of him. Ironically we retired on the same amount of games, 192. Injuries, suspensions and such made up the difference.

Even though it was my first game, I was played for the four quarters. I'm not ashamed to admit, I was scared. I was small, and from what I can recall of that game, it was really rough. It was absolutely frightening. Bondy was about the same size as me but he was a ferocious little bugger and had a reputation of really getting stuck into you. He was pretty good to me though, knowing I was young, but it was definitely very physical. The other huge difference was the fans. Going from WAFL games, which had several thousand fans at best, to about 20,000-25,000 fans was a massive thing to get used to. The fans were abusive to the team and to me, because I looked so young. They were yelling out *"go back to school"* and all that sort of thing. The crowd intimidated me that first year, there's no doubt about that.

The worst game for fans in that first year was at Victoria Park, which was Collingwood's home ground. Fans would throw empty VB tins at you. I had an empty four-litre sauce bottle thrown over the fence at me. Our bench seats were set among the normal seats and the crowd could touch you if they wanted. They didn't, but they were right there in your ear with *"you little poof"*, *"homo"* and more. When I think back, now, it was pretty heavy stuff for a teenager to have to put up with.

In terms of the footy, going from Victorian Under-17s, to a few games in the WAFL, then to AFL were just huge steps. WAFL and the AFL may have the same rules but they are worlds apart in intensity, speed and how you are tackled. AFL is bigger and faster. The ball travels from one end of the ground to the other quicker than any other league and the intensity of body and mental pressure is phenomenal. I was tackled, harassed and pummelled for the entirely of a game. I tried my guts out, and never gave in but at the end of the day I was exhausted.

Once I had been in the AFL ranks for some time and found myself dropped back to the WAFL, it was actually a very relaxing time. There was still the expectation to perform, very much so, but it was more relaxed from the time you left your house through to the warm-up. When I played at AFL level, the meetings were more precise, the theory and tactics to break down the opposition more intense and it continued right through the week leading up to the game. The coach might ask the team to watch a huge amount of video through the week to break down the opponent's strengths, or to watch a video on an individual opponent you are going to play on. That really didn't happen at WAFL level.

Then there was the issue of travel. Back then, we used to fly to the East coast the day before the game, which was no good. We would fly in the morning, leave Perth at about 11am get in at 5pm, go straight to the hotel, stretch, have dinner, and go to bed. Because I was a bad flier, I was always exhausted. You'd have to deal with the travel and time change then play at 2.10pm the next day. The West coast-based teams were really ripped off in that way back then. Nowadays, if you are playing a Saturday game, you would leave Thursday and have a couple of days to train, relax, prepare, and get over jet lag. The only way I can describe travel back then to people is like playing with a hangover. Of course, it was all to do with money. The AFL would only pay for one night's accommodation, and the club couldn't afford for us to stay that extra night, but things are different now.

As well as changes in travel, the whole financial set-up and payments to players have improved over the years. Back when I started, because I was a top 20 draft pick, I got an extra bonus, but the base payment for a first year player was $20,000 guaranteed. I was paid $1500 per senior grade game, so I actually made $28,000 in my first year for playing 15 games. With bonuses, you might make $3000 in bonus payments for playing four AFL games; maybe $5000 for eight AFL games and $7500 for 15 AFL games. Fremantle paid Theresa for my board in the first year and gave her extra money to cook, clean, iron and so on. The only expense I had was fuel for my car, my mobile phone and entertainment. So in my first year with all those bonuses, I grossed about $90,000. For an 18-year-old back in 1997, that was huge money, big bucks.

My second match was against St Kilda at Subiaco and I kicked two goals, which was a big deal. Back then, it was really intimidating for a visiting team to come to Subiaco Oval because at the eastern end, behind the goals, there was no seating, just a grassy slope. The Freo diehards used to sit there and play bongo drums for the whole game. The bongos are now banned, but it proved just how committed and unique Fremantle fans could be. For me in my second match, it just added to the flavour of the whole game and gave me a taste of what was to come.

I was nominated for the Norwich Rising Star Award, which is now known as the NAB AFL Rising Star. It is like the Brownlow Medal for first year players. I didn't win it but it was great to be nominated. My second match also stands out for me because I was fortunate enough to play on Robert Harvey, who I later played with at St Kilda. He was an idol of mine. He went on to win the Brownlow Medal that year and was about five leagues above everyone else and really impressive to watch and to play on. But rather than intimidate me, playing on Harvs brought out my best. Later in my career at Freo, coach Chris Connolly would always play me on Harvs. Even then, when he was older, he used to run so hard. He was an amazing athlete, a great bloke and a dual Brownlow medallist (1997-1998). He retired the same year as me at the age of 38, having played nearly 400 games.

The standouts of my first year were my first game against Richmond, the Norwich Rising Star nomination and the fact I played most of the games, most of the time, all the way to the last game of Round 22 in the AFL. I also played in the winning South Fremantle team against arch rivals East Fremantle in the WAFL grand final that year. I ended up with about 26 touches and played well in front of 38,000 people, which, at the time, was the biggest crowd I had ever played for. It was one of those great moments of my career. It ended up being the only senior grand final I played in and won, and it was in just my first year of footy. Can you believe it? I thought, this is all too easy, bring it on!

It was a fairytale, but the next year, 1998, I was struck down by injury and only played one match. In the industry, this is put down to what we call the 'Footy Gods'. They are up there somewhere, waiting to take it away from you as quickly as they gave it to you. I think Malcolm Blight – who was a champion player and coach – came up with that one, but I tend to agree with him. Footy as a career is like a roller coaster.

CHAPTER 7
FEAR AND LOATHING

"It seems I was co-dependent on chaos to perform, and consciously, or subconsciously, associated success, or being the best I could be, with a chaotic world."

That first year in the AFL was brilliant, but as the years went by, playing with the Dockers and St Kilda, my anxiety grew worse. I would get extremely anxious going to public places. I didn't realise there was anything wrong with me because I had always been dealing with some type of anxiety ever since I was a kid. What I certainly didn't realise was that the experience was not uncommon among AFL players.

People would be shocked at how many AFL players are on some type of medication. The year I retired I wasn't the only player on anti-depressants; in fact several of my team mates confided in me that they were taking them and I wouldn't be surprised if there were more I didn't know about. I think that would most likely have applied to all clubs in the AFL. I'm sure the public would wonder why, but for me, the answer is simple. I think the public perceives footballers as some kind of 'supermen', especially when they see us on the field, but in actual fact when you break down an AFL player's mental state he is far from that. Every team has a full-time psychologist, constantly working with each player to get the best out of him and to help him conquer his fears. One of the biggest fears for me was the fear of failure; of not succeeding on that huge stage called a football field.

In some way, every single AFL footballer has to be the most selfish person on the planet because to make it onto a list you have to be completely egocentric. However, once you get on the list it changes, it's all about being a team player; to get the best out of yourself, to do the best for the team. This is where the conflict lies and what plays havoc with your mental state. It's a constant battle of knowing what works for you from a self-centred point of view, and balancing that with what's best for the team.

For example, your coach may ask you to tag a player and shut him out of the game, even though this mightn't be natural to your game. It's what's best for the team. It's hard to describe – the best way is sort of Jekyll and Hyde. If you succeed for the team that week and do your job, that's great from the coach's point of view but from a personal point of view it might make you feel vulnerable.

One of my main anxiety drivers was my fear of flying. A fear I've had since I was a child. I used to suffer a lot when I had to get on an airplane. It was mainly due to feeling I wasn't in control, and I was also frightened of crashing. If I had been flying the plane, I would have been as cool as a cucumber. As you can imagine, I was a mess travelling to and from interstate football matches. I would have to drink about four litres of water to hydrate before getting on the plane because I would sweat unbelievably. It would just pour out of me. It was a really hard time because I didn't recognise it as anxiety, I just thought I had a fear of flying and that was it.

I used to deny the fear and say to myself, *"you're a grown man, you're in your Fremantle gear, and people are watching, pull yourself together"*. All my teammates knew what I was going through but they just gave me shit, especially when we went through turbulence. I would hold onto the chair or I'd grab one of my teammate's legs. One time I was in the aisle seat and we were coming back into Perth. It was terrible weather and I was exhausted from the game, which made my anxiety worse. It was bumpy for about an hour and I was trembling, tapping my legs and holding the seat the whole time. One of my teammates sitting close started saying, *"oh, no Blacky, we're going to crash, we're going to crash"*. That really didn't help.

I spoke to club psychologists and it helped a bit, but I still used to struggle with it. I remember another time I got on the plane and my core temperature felt like it went up 100 degrees and I nearly fainted. I couldn't breathe, so instead of calling for help, knowing all my mates would just have a go, I unlocked my seat belt, got up and ran to the toilet. I just covered myself in water and I sat on the toilet while the stewards were banging on the door because the plane was waiting to take off. When I came out all the boys were looking at me and shaking their heads.

BLACK

While I was a professional footballer there were times I got myself into trouble in public purely because of my anxiety.

One particular time, I was in the Clink nightclub in Fremantle and had just walked in with a couple of other football players and some other friends. I was coming down the stairs and I had a panic attack. No one would have even known what was going on, but I had this overwhelming feeling that I didn't want to be there. I was overheating and could hardly breathe. My response to the panic was to smash down as many drinks as quickly as I could until I loosened up.

Initially that was fine, but later on in the evening, I became very tense. I got into a push-and-shove with a patron, but was able to get into a backroom and take off and get away with it. This wasn't the first or the last time something like this would happen. Over time I could see a pattern of this sort of thing emerging. I recognise now I feel uncomfortable being around strangers and meeting new people. It makes me anxious and can bring out the worst in me, especially if I've been drinking.

Getting myself into these situations only put more pressure on me. I thought I was an extremely team-oriented person, I certainly was on the field, but I let myself down off the field with the things I did. I'd say to myself *"you represent the club, but here you are fighting with strangers"*. But then I would turn it around in my own head to justify my behaviour.

FEAR AND LOATHING

There were other players like me who starting drinking and rebelling during the week, both at Fremantle and St Kilda. I suppose we are what some would call 'blokey blokes'. We'd pull a chair out for a woman to sit down, open the door and let her walk through first, that sort of stuff. Socially we were the larrikins, the life of the party, with our mates; strong, we'd demand respect. I'd gravitate towards these types of people, they were my mates. We recognised that we were a little bit different and not like the AFL mould; the robot mould that the team wanted. Mind you, despite that behaviour off the footy field, once we crossed that white boundary line, we were often the six most important players on the ground.

Perhaps in my era, players could get away with the shenanigans during the week, but I don't think it's the case now. The game has become too fast and you just can't afford to do what we used to do leading up to a game. Whether that is drinking, or lack of sleep or eating a kebab. What you see now in the AFL, are players who are more disciplined but, to my mind, lack personality. I feel sorry for this new breed of players. They can't be themselves and their whole life is consumed by trying to do the right thing by the team and by the coaches. They can't socialise and, if they do, they get fined. They're told when to drink, when to eat; just about when to wipe their arse. It was tough for us, but it's much tougher now.

Looking back, I think it was this 'blokey' thing that got in the way of an earlier diagnosis of my Bipolar II. Dad raised me with a strong concept of what a man is supposed to be and I was very influenced by some of Dad's younger friends, who were very hard, hard men.

I was still playing AFL when I finally worked out there was something wrong with me, that the whole blokey thing wasn't cutting it, and that I needed some help. It was a couple of years before the end of my career when I got on to the Beyond Blue website and I looked up anxiety and did their survey: I ticked nearly every bloody box! I rang the AFL Players' Association (AFLPA), our players' union, and spoke to the head psychologist. After checking me out, they absolutely supported me.

The AFLPA is great and in this case I felt like I could go to them before my club. I was so excited about finding a solution to my anxiety. The club gave me permission to take a small amount of sleeping pills, which made things a lot better. The tablets made me relax within half an hour of taking them, which would in turn take away the fear and many of the anxiety symptoms. They worked for my fear of flying as well as the night before games to help me get a good night's sleep. I called it my wonder drug. Upon reflection I should have been taking something like that from day dot, but I just never knew what anxiety was, I just saw my behaviour as a weakness. The only other time I felt the same calmness was when I drank alcohol. Obviously on the plane or just before a match, this was not an option.

At the time, putting a name to my condition was a huge relief. I found I could look back through my life and understand why I did this or that, as well as understand the way I was feeling. I now realise, though, that the medication

I was on for two years was wrong and really just a Band-Aid. It's hard to say, but I sometimes wonder if I would have had a couple more years of top level footy in me if things had been different. Sure the body was starting to deteriorate but what it really came down to was that, mentally, I was out of it and in the end I just couldn't get away from the game quick enough. Don't get me wrong, I don't blame anyone for this and I'm certainly not bitter about my career being over prematurely, it's just food for thought.

To be honest, I don't know how someone with my make-up survived in an elite sport at all. I ended up not loving football, in fact, I probably only loved it for the first two or three years of AFL, then the next 10 years were a pain in the arse. I kept doing it because it was good money; I loved the camaraderie and got a natural high from the euphoria associated with winning. But it wasn't enough to stop it from becoming a grind, it became a real effort because of my mental state. I just wasn't aware of what was happening inside myself. I was always in self-destruct mode. When things were going well I would toe the line during the week, play football and then hit the self-destruct button and just go mental drinking after the game.

It seems I was co-dependent on chaos to perform, and consciously, or subconsciously, associated success, or being the best I could be, with a chaotic world. I was dealing with the extremes of massive highs and massive lows. I actually had artwork for a tattoo made up around this time of my life, which I haven't used. It is of three people on a roller coaster, each in their own separate carriage. One carriage is on its way up the track, the next one is balancing on top of the track and the third is coming down the other side. Little did I know then, but the tattoo sums up Bipolar II perfectly: massive highs and lows are all part of the condition. In the old days they used to call it manic depression. That was me before I got on the right medication, and certainly in all the years I played professional football – either manic or depressed.

CHAPTER 8
A LOSING STREAK AT THE GALLOPS

"My friends didn't understand what I was going through. I didn't understand myself. They just thought I was a nut. My behaviour suddenly changed. I went from being one person to another, instantly. My friends just thought it was Blacky being Blacky. Looking back, that's exactly what Bipolar II is all about, but I didn't know it at the time."

A very public example of my extreme behaviour was one New Year's Day at the race track for the Perth Cup. A lot has been said in the media about that ugly incident when I was charged with assault occasioning bodily harm, obstructing police and assaulting a female police officer.

Google me and you'll find a reference about the Perth Cup under my name in Wikipedia. It states that there was talk that I was going to change my name to Heath Purple as part of a promotion with Ribena, but *"it may have been cancelled because of the charges"*. I'll set the record straight now – there never was going to be a Heath Purple and after that shocker of a day, it would have been the last thing on my mind.

So here's the actual true story for what it's worth. It's not pretty. It's not an excuse, but it was at a time before I'd been diagnosed with any type of mental condition and I was in a dark, dark place.

I was really looking forward to going to the Perth Cup. I hadn't gone out the night before because my anxiety was always worse when I was really looking forward to something. I did that once and never made that mistake again. I remember going to the Red Hot Chili Peppers' concert, and I had been looking forward to going to it for ages. The day of the concert arrived and I decided to drive all my mates in, stone cold sober, because I was scared of going. They had all started drinking before we got there, but I just didn't feel well enough to do it. My friends didn't understand what I was going through. I didn't understand myself. They just thought I was a nut. My behaviour suddenly changed. I went from being one person to another, instantly. My friends just thought it was Blacky being Blacky. Looking back, that's exactly what Bipolar II is all about, but I didn't know it at the time.

The Perth Cup was a really big deal for me because my brothers were coming over from Melbourne. I was still with the Dockers at the time, we'd had a good year, everything was going well, but my anxiety leading up to the Perth Cup was overwhelming. I nearly didn't go – I didn't want to go, but I did. We got there and I was really anxious, I had diarrhoea before I went, was feeling sick in the stomach and was generally unwell, but I pushed on. I had two beers in the car on the way and it was all pretty much a binge drinking fiesta from there on in. Anyone who has ever been to the Perth Cup would know what it was like. It was hot and back then there were unlimited drinks, and we all got hammered really quickly – everyone was extremely pissed. I was in a tent with a lot of other AFL players and everyone was kicked out because there was supposedly some bar staff handing out drugs. I was with my brother, other AFL players, which from memory didn't include any Freo players, some media identities and a few celebrities.

Finally we were allowed back in the tent, and we were just doing our thing, when the beer ran out. What they did, which is illegal now, was to make up 10 litre drums of bourbon and coke and vodka and lemonade and people were lining up with plastic cups, walking past and scooping up grog. That's how feral it was. Then that ran out. We had paid big bucks and everyone was shitty, so we decided to get these two litre bottles of spirits and just slammed them down, passing it around to whoever was nearby. We got the grog from anywhere we could, there were tents everywhere.

We were all very, very drunk.

Then my 17-year-old brother Dean went missing. Like the rest of us, he was extremely pissed but he was in my care. He wasn't meant to be there because he was 17, so I knew there was a danger, so we went to look for him. It was towards the end of the day and we were being asked to leave.

I rang him on his mobile and he was incoherent; I couldn't understand what he was saying or where he was. I thought he kept hanging up, but in fact he was falling asleep. We worked out he was way down at another entrance, but we still couldn't find him. It didn't help that I was pole axed. It's Perth Cup and alcohol was my drug of choice at the time, but the level of drunkenness was way up there.

Dean later told me the following series of events took place when he went 'missing'.

A bloke walked up and asked him for a cigarette, but Dean told him he didn't smoke. The guy said *"give me a cigarette"*; again, *"I don't smoke"*. Anyway it was a bit of a set-up. My brother was sitting down, the other guy was standing up and the bloke just whacked him, unprovoked. Dean is quite a good brawler, solid like me so he retaliated. He attacked this guy who was a lot older, about 25, and started to get on top of him. Then five more of this dickhead's mates came and kicked the shit out of Dean. He ended up with a broken nose and completely beaten up – they gave him the works.

Then I finally found him. I hadn't seen anything that had happened I just found him and he was a mess, his nose was across his face and the guys had gone. He gave me a rough description of his attackers and I sent my brother-in-law to the left and I went the other way and I just said *"seek and destroy"*.

We didn't find them and Dean needed medical attention so we decided to leave. I had tears coming down my face I was so angry. Just then I got some shit from a guy who recognised me as an AFL player. He asked me what I was crying about, and I told him to *"fuck off"*. I started running to get out of there and then I slowed. I thought I saw the people Dean had described to me as his attackers. Right then a random bloke hip and shouldered me, a random person, but I just turned around and slapped him with an open hand. I smacked him instinctively as hard as I could and the force knocked him out for six minutes. That one open handed smack broke his collar bone.

He went down and it triggered a fit of blind rage in me. I was so wound up I was even thinking about attacking this guy's friends even though all they were doing was trying to help him. The rage passed and my senses started to come back and my first reaction was to get out of there. I started running in a different direction but by then the police had arrived and so I just started fighting them too. God, I don't know why, it was all so fast and crazy. The female police officer came in from my right where I couldn't see her, so I didn't know who it was. I just felt a hand on my back and I automatically turned around and pushed. Over she went.

My immediate thought was *"oh shit"*. I knew I was in a lot of trouble. Not only had I pushed a police officer, and I have the utmost respect for the coppers, it was a woman. The male officers converged and did I finally back down? No, I was out of control. I just started fighting them, heaps of them, probably five. I punched a couple and then finally I started to get my senses back and tried to calm down. I said *"all right, all right"*, and got down on my knees. They gave me a good flogging, but you know what, I deserved it. One of the coppers flipped me over while I was being arrested and dropped his knee into my sternum. A couple of days later I had to go to the doctor and get a cracked rib looked at. I don't blame the coppers, good on them, I was a drunken maniac.

I can't describe how I felt at the time. I had never felt like that before. I have never had an experience where a loved one, a brother, was hurt like that. What happened later in Bali was a similar incident where I thought my brother was in danger and something in me just snapped.

If I had been sober I would have worked through it all a lot better and I definitely would not have fought with the police or pushed a female officer. I apologised to her straight away. I remember actually getting arrested, and saying *"stop, stop, stop, I have the utmost respect for you, I am really, really sorry"*. I've subsequently apologised in public. My main regret, which still plays on my mind, is that we never actually found the guy involved with bashing Dean. He got away with turning my baby brother's face into a bloody pulp. I know I should let it go, but it still enrages me to this day.

There was a lock-up facility at the Perth Cup and that's where they put me. After a while they released me and I went home, but the next day they came to my house and arrested me, taking me to the Armadale Police Station to be fingerprinted. I had the book thrown at me, and it showed me how easy it was to find myself on the wrong side of the law. I have been to Casuarina Prison to play footy matches with the prisoners as a community service, and I found that a bit scary, but it was probably good for me to see what a scary place prison is. It opened my eyes to a whole other world and what might have been for me.

The person I hit never pressed charges but I was charged by the police with assault occasioning bodily harm, which is a jail term if convicted. I was also charged with assaulting a public officer and obstructing police. I think they let me off lightly with the charges, I reckon I could have gone for two assaults on public officers, especially the male officer. There was a long drawn out court process and I ended up being fined $5000. The club could have fined me an extra $5000, but they didn't, they thought I had been punished enough after five or six appearances in court, each time with TV cameras shoved in my face. The whole process took a year and I felt I was certainly punished enough. It was a horrible thing to go through.

Had I learnt my lesson? No. Did that get me kicked out of the AFL? No. The Perth Cup incident didn't spell the end of my career, far from it. I kept playing for the Dockers and my problems with anxiety and anger only got worse. My addiction to grog only got worse. I was becoming more and more out of control.

That railway carriage was careening down the tracks at a frightening rate of knots.

CHAPTER 9
THE DEMON DRINK

"All the occasions I have been in trouble with the law, have always involved alcohol; I have never ever gotten into trouble, sober."

It should have been pretty obvious to me and those around me that I was not coping with life. Even though I had lost my passion for the game, I still always gave everything I had for the jumper, the team and the supporters. But little did the fans know that when I was walking up the race before coming on to the ground at the start of each game, I would often vomit because of the anxiety. Before the game we would have our second warm-up and we would have six minutes to run in and get changed. About four minutes of that six, I would quickly run in and put on my 'Superman suit' (uniform) and run straight to the toilet. I would be sitting there sweating and go through this process of trying to calm myself down.

The other boys would all be warming up, stretching, and hitting bags. All I was doing – and I'm not even very religious – was praying. I just asked whoever was listening to help me get through the next two hours of my life because it felt like the hardest thing to cope with. I even vomited on Shaunie Mac's legs once before a West Coast game. You ask anyone, I used to vomit all the time. I'd be dry retching in the huddles. Everyone was pretty much used to it, but during one final when we were playing in Adelaide, one of the guys came up to me and told me to get a grip. It was our first final so I was all over the shop but I ended up getting best-on-ground with about 36 touches.

My anxiety was debilitating in so many ways but I used to use the way I felt as a real positive, making that fear of failure a motivation to perform. When the game was over it was a huge relief. There was a sense of joy, and if we won and played well, it was the best feeling ever. Then when that night was over, it was back to the grindstone and the anxiety would return and by Wednesday I'd be back to vomiting.

I played in two preliminary finals – one with St Kilda and one with Freo. I often think about whether it would have been better to live the dream of playing in an AFL Grand Final or if I was happy we lost the preliminary final so I didn't have to go through the hell of a grand final week. I don't know how I would have reacted if my team had played in a grand final. I reckon I would have been reported for sure because I would've gone nuts. I was always among the best players during finals, so it seemed I performed well when the stakes were high and the anxiety grew.

To compound my mental issues, I was addicted to alcohol. It was both my crutch and my albatross. I thought it helped me cope but it didn't help at all. In fact it added fuel to the fire. There were rules about drinking while you played in the AFL, but most of the time I didn't give a shit about the rules, I just drank. I would drink on Monday during the football season, going to the pub and having between six and 20 beers depending on how I felt. I was very single-minded and selfish off the field, but around the club and on the field, I always tried to be a real team player. This link between sport and drinking was a strong one for me as it is with many Australians, and, like most Aussies, our footy 'celebrations' often involved large amounts of alcohol.

MAD MONDAYS

One annual event which involved a lot of drinking was Mad Mondays. Someone told me recently that Mad Mondays were no longer endorsed by the AFL. Back when I played, Mad Mondays were a very traditional day where the team got together and everyone just got drunk. It happened at the end of the year, whenever the team finished. So if it was a Saturday night match, and your team was out of the finals, you would have a function on Saturday night after the game, and then go out and get hammered, the wives and partners included.

At St Kilda it was extremely organised, which I think was probably for the best because when the club was involved they could monitor exactly what went on. One year we played at the Telstra Dome in Melbourne, so we went to the function room to celebrate the end of the year. Sponsors and other VIPs were invited and there were about 200-300 people in the room.

Win or lose, for the footy players it's the end of their year. If your team hadn't made the finals then you were upset but glad the year was over. On the other side of the coin, if your team was in the finals and lost, of course, you were extra upset and, although it was the last thing you felt like doing, it was compulsory to attend the function. It was usual to stay for an hour or so, which meant about eight beers for me. I used to get right into it.

In this environment I knew I had to do my bit and then get out of there real quick. I suppose that was for a couple of reasons. If we'd had an unsuccessful year and people were coming up saying *"better luck next year"* that was OK, but it never went down well when people started telling me what I could do better, or where my team went wrong. I would give them their five minutes of fame and then go to the toilet, or get a drink or something, simple as that. If we'd just lost a final or a preliminary final, it would be more about reminiscing over the year. It was always a bit easier if we had been beaten on the day by a quality team – then you just had to deal with it. During my professional career I lost two preliminary finals, which was tough.

Really though, I often just wanted to get out of there. I'd drink quite heavily because it was free alcohol, but then I'd just wanted to wind up the year with my teammates. In my later years, I was an organiser of the 'after after' parties but even when I was about 20, I organised a huge show at Moondyne Joe's in Fremantle. About 600 supporters and players turned up. That sort of show's not done much anymore. It is too much money, too political and not acceptable. Football is now big business and you can't afford to have a major slip up on the piss. The media are on to it and the sponsors are watching.

I don't like the way it is going but I understand why, and with my reputation, who am I to talk? It had just got to the stage where too many people had fucked up and it was no longer acceptable in anyone's eyes.

FOOTY TRIPS

The other big opportunity for drinking and carrying on like a pork chop was, of course, the footy trips. Everyone has a view on footy trips. I know lots of people who can't come to terms with the fact that an elite sportsman, a famous person, can go overseas and fuck as many girls as he wants, and then he comes back and all is normal. The players used to raise money throughout the year for the end-of-season trip, through functions, cinema nights and so on. One year the whole team signed 100 Dockers jumpers and sold them for $250 each. The players would have a trip contribution taken out of our pays every month. A trip like this would cost about $100,000. It was serious stuff.

What I have now heard through the grapevine is that the clubs have removed themselves from these footy trips and don't endorse them. But for all of my AFL footy career it was endorsed. We had a chaperone who was nominated to stay reasonably sober and keep an eye on everyone. The club did qualify the role of the chaperone – he provided the first aid, he could drink but not much; he was not one of the team and he was always a guy.

In the late 90s we went to the Gold Coast for one trip. One night I got back to the hotel at about 4am, smashed. The boys were still drinking piss and going nuts. We turned the lights off and started to wrestle, and one of the guys hit his head on the corner of the bedside table and knocked himself out cold. I had to wake the chaperone up to sort it out.

By then the player, who will remain anonymous, had woken and we couldn't control him. He was extremely pissed, I think he had about 20 shots of vodka, so he was going nuts, and he was a big boy. Anyway we threw him in the bath and ran cold water over him and got him to wake up properly. He was in his jocks, which got him very, very upset. So the chaperone calmed him down, while we all continued drinking. The player then decided that he wanted to go home. The problem was we were 18 storeys up and we certainly didn't want him taking the quick way down. He did find his way out onto the balcony but we weren't having any of that so I said to the boys *"I've gotta get him back inside, so I'm going to knock him out again"*. I ran out and dragged him to the ground on the balcony and just absolutely punched him straight in the head. So once again he was pretty much out to the world. What else could I do? He could've killed himself. He missed his plane the next day and still hasn't thanked me to this day. Funny that.

Crazy things happened on the footy trips all the time. I don't think we actually lost anyone, but I came close myself

THE DEMON DRINK

once on our footy trip to Thailand in 2008, the year I retired. I went to a club with some of the younger boys and was carrying on like a tosser making disrespectful comments for all to hear. As it turns out some of these comments were about the owner's wife. He'd heard what I had said and came up and said, *"I'm going to shoot you"*. He then pulled a gun out of his pocket and pointed it at me. I just turned around and said *"whatever, mate"*.

The boys I was with gave me no support, they just ran once they saw the gun, that was it, they were off. So I was left to my own devices, and luckily I just walked away.

I ended up in Shantytown about 15km way out the back of Phuket in the hills, and it was pissing with rain. I don't know how I ended up there, walked I suppose, but these locals, they go *"hey Superman, Superman, you big boy, you big boy, come, come drink"*. So I sat with them drinking their own home concoction listening to them play guitar. I was on my own and I had been drunk for three days straight, so I was way past it all. I woke up the next day still in Shantytown with just a pair of shorts on, no shirt, no nothing, and sleeping with the whole family on one mattress. There were 20 of them in there. My kidneys were still intact, thank God, but in the cold light of day, it was pretty hairy.

During that entire trip, I was in a really bad place. We had a rule that if we went out on our own, we would meet back at a certain point every night at six to make sure everyone was OK and still alive. Well, at times, I didn't even turn up for that and even though I would cop a bollocking for it, I didn't care. The older blokes were like, *"Blacky, you are out of control"*. I just told them to *"fuck off"*. My self-destruction had already begun.

I had my anxiety and depression medication with me in Thailand and those five days saw me take the most number of tablets I've ever taken in my life. I was popping that many anti-depressants and drinking that heavily I would push right through, pass out, wake up to go to the toilet, and then not go back to sleep. So to combat that mania and try to get some rest, I would take massive amounts of sleeping pills. I spent the whole trip popping some form of prescription medication and drinking ... what a fucking mess.

The gun incident proved something to me – I thought I was invincible. I couldn't have given two shits if someone wanted to attack me, I was actually nearing the stage where I wanted it to happen, so I could get hurt to the point where I no longer had to face things. Maybe even be killed. I had never felt like that before. I just wanted something to get me out of the pain of what I was going through. Of course I did take it to the next level a few months later in Bali.

CHAPTER 10
THE LIGHT AT THE END

"Some people called me Jekyll and Hyde, while Asha called my different personalities Heath and *Keith*. Actually it was more than Jekyll and Hyde or Heath and *Keith*; there was a whole bloody team of people inside me."

My rapid downfall began after retirement at the end of 2008, which continued to gain momentum until the end of 2009. Some of the events of that year are outlined earlier, but Asha tells the story as she saw it in Chapter 12. Reading her story is like a knife in my guts every time.

After my diagnosis for Bipolar II and going onto new medication at the start of 2010, I finally got a break. I was given a job with BCE Surveying as a surveyor's assistant and also as the head coach of Harvey Brunswick Leschenault Football Club in the south west of Western Australia – go the Lions! I was honest with them and they gave me a crack when no one else was interested.

Asha and I moved from Northbridge to a small coastal community and life started to find some normality, especially away from the world of AFL football. Getting the job and living and working in a small community were the best things that could have happened, especially acquiring a lower profile.

I'm no superstar, but Perth people love footballers and football certainly opened many doors for me. But it's a double-edged sword. You get opportunities but people just use you for what you do, not who you are. I began feeling indebted to those people who gave me these opportunities and I went well beyond the call of duty to satisfy their requests. I felt almost subservient. As a consequence, I was finding myself in environments that really weren't suited to my state of mind and, thinking about it, probably fed the demon within. It was all self-inflicted mind you, but it wasn't a healthy place to be.

Moving to the country and getting away from all the madness gave me time to reflect and learn more about myself. One thing I came to realise, which seems so clear now, is that I am just not comfortable being around people I don't know. It's hard to define, but walking into a crowded area, be it a pub or a music festival, I feel intimidated by all the people I don't know. More than intimidated, actually, I feel threatened. I don't want to meet or talk to anyone. To take it one step further, it makes me anxious when I am approached by a stranger, male or female. I just don't know what they are going to ask or do.

For example, in mid-2010, a state newspaper wrote an article about me, including a photo. The day it came out, I was sitting in my car with my two sons waiting for Asha to come out of the chemist, when I was approached by two tough looking guys who tapped on the car window. It's hard to explain the feelings that went through me. I felt instantly that this was only going to go one of two ways – they were either going to say *"how are you going, mate?"* or they were going to have a go. I just wanted to get out of there. I was scared of how I would react and what they would do.

I decided to open the door and said a stern hello. This is where it kind of gets funny. They said *"you're Simon Black aren't you?"*. Simon is actually a Brisbane Lions' player who is a Brownlow medallist, so I was pretty happy to be put in his category. Immediately I knew they were footy fans, if not slightly ill-informed ones, and told them my name was Heath Black. After they got over their embarrassment, one asked for an autograph on the back of his pay slip for his mum, Chookie.

It turned out fine, but I had immediately flown into a state where I was ready to defend myself and my boys. It brought on all the symptoms of anxiety – heart-thumping, core-body temperature going through the roof, lack of breath, muscles contracting, jaw clenching – that then flicked into anger almost immediately. The reaction is out of my control, it all depends on the stranger and where they are coming from. I'm like an animal ready to attack if provoked. This incident ended up in laughter, but my boys still don't understand why people are so intrusive.

By the time Asha got back to the car, I'd calmed down, but she sensed something had happened. Asha had become my counsellor and, as usual, as I debriefed on what had just happened, it seemed so small, but it wasn't. It's what I used to go through all the time, except this time it didn't come to blows.

I'm trying hard to control the beast brought on by Bipolar II. It's a strange animal though. It can lay dormant then be triggered by a major life event – in my case retiring from the AFL and my previous marriage breaking up. No one knows how long I might have suffered from the condition. Even when I played footy in the Under-9s, I was an aggressive little shit. When I spoke to Mum after the diagnosis, she thought that I hadn't been quite right for a while. She said to me *"I always knew you were a little different"*. She thought it was ADHD and because there were not so many solutions around when I was a kid, she just focused on getting me to expend my energy playing sport.

I think football was a natural medication for my Bipolar II and when it was taken away there was no escape from all the extremes.

THE MANY FACES OF HEATH

Some people called me Jekyll and Hyde, while Asha called my different personalities Heath and *Keith*. Actually it was more than Jekyll and Hyde or Heath and *Keith*; there was a whole bloody team of people inside of me. Asha and I worked out I had about four different personality types which came out depending on the situation.

There was Heath 1, the man Asha fell in love with and the man I want to be. Heath 1 is loving, caring and giving to her and others. He is a caring Dad who puts his kids first, plays with them, encourages them and is completely engrossed in their company. Being on the medication and not drinking helps bring this man to the fore.

Heath 2 (or *Keith*) is the opposite and often comes out when I'm drunk. He's a knock-about chauvinistic arsehole, who is disrespectful to women, flirts in front of Asha and is usually seen when I am around other footballers.

Heath 3 is a politician. This Heath was very useful in my football career. I had the ability to do old-fashioned networking, work people out and see what pushed their buttons. This used to make me feel powerful, especially if I could outwit an educated person who thought they were better than me. When I was Heath 3, I always felt like I had something to prove. Finally there was Heath 4, the salesman who loved to bullshit.

Can you imagine how hard it was to live like that? Or in Asha's case, live with that sort of person? Thank God for medication.

I'm now on Xanax, or my magic little pill as Asha calls it. It helps me straight away. I pop one under my tongue and it blocks all the anxiety, takes away the feelings of nervousness, calms my heart rate, stops the worrying thoughts, and stops the paranoia. Asha's had some experiences in her life that have equipped her to see through my charade, but it took a while after my diagnosis for her to accept my mental illness. She finally believed me, forgave me for my actions and has completely supported me to get back on track. She can assess my mood at a glance and knows whether I'm capable of handling a situation or if we need to leave. I now keep a mood diary that helps me analyse my moods.

Although I'd like to say otherwise, it's not all been smooth sailing since I've lived down south. One day in mid-2010, in my role as head football coach of the local team, we had a social occasion at our house. Two of the players started mucking around inside, just play fighting really, then jumping up and touching the ceiling. They grabbed one of the trophies and smashed it on ground and something in me just snapped. Fists were thrown but suddenly I realised what I was doing. I managed to just stop and walk away. In the past that would never have happened. I would have just kept banging away until someone restrained me.

Despite me leaving, it turned into a real ugly event in Bunbury. I found I was falling back into some old depressive habits. That night at the brewery I'd been binge drinking, a huge no-no for me. People stopped talking to us and I thought the only solution was to quit my job. I started questioning the diagnosis and the medication, but then I looked at it more deeply and I realised I had let my medication slip. I had started to backslide into old patterns. I just can't do that, I need to stick to guidelines. Thank God my footy team won the grand final – the local community was prepared to give me one more shot.

But I decided something else then too. It was time to draw a line in the sand with people – it's OK if they don't like me but like anyone else, I deserve some respect and consistency. Don't prance around the big AFL player and pretend he's your mate, then drop him like a hot potato at the first sign of trouble. Looking back at it all I still wonder who I really am. So do my family and loved ones.

To this day I believe my step-Dad, Mum and Dad still don't really believe I have Bipolar II. First up they think I'm lying because of all the excuses I have subjected them and others to. I've also been known to exaggerate a story or two. And I think it might be difficult for people of their generation to accept mental illness. Some people have asked me why I care what my family thinks. I mean, I've been away from them since I was 17. But I am still close to my family and despite the distance from WA to Victoria I've always stayed in close contact.

I started writing this story in the middle of 2009 at the crisis point of my life. I then shelved it while I worked through the many challenges I had created for myself. It was only recently that Asha and I discussed the book coming out of the bottom drawer. It's a risk for me coming back 'out' in the public arena, and I wasn't sure how I was going to cope. I was nervous about the return of salesman Heath, fuelled by the attention of the media, text messages and emails from people who don't know me, wanting to be my best friend again.

Writing this book, for me, has been about educating people, not about feeding my ego. I don't need or want the publicity. I'm busy living my life and trying to be Heath 1. The one thing I do want is for my sons, Chayce and Cayden, to understand me. If they Google me and see what's on the web, what are they going to think? I don't want them to grow up thinking their Dad is a dickhead. I hope it's not too late.

Nowadays I am more structured and more reliable; I can reason out things. The depressive thoughts and anxiety have taken a back seat, which is an amazing feeling. I'm happier now than I was, but I know that the demons could easily reappear. It's about being vigilant and staying away from temptation, which is a daily challenge for me. What gets me through is my vision of a future with Asha, surrounded by family in a safe, happy place where I can ultimately find peace.

CHAPTER 11
RING OF FIRE

"My deep-lying passion, and the reason I am in the public arena, speaking to people, is that I believe my story may help prevent a suicide, or stop a person ending up in jail, or from hurting someone. It may stop someone from drink-driving and injuring themselves or someone else. Or it may simply stop the destruction of a relationship."

Just when you think you've found the solution, that you're on track, getting better, whatever that might mean, you can feel your gut telling you something is still missing. After finding out I had Bipolar II and was on the 'right' medication I still felt something was missing. It was like I was 90 per cent there but 10 per cent wasn't quite right.

I revealed to the world my diagnosis of Bipolar II at the Men in Black Ball in Perth in June 2011. Dr John Clarkson heard me speak at the ball and invited me to come and visit him to have a chat. To cut a long story short, on top of

Bipolar II, I have been diagnosed with a classic case of Adult ADHD Type 6.

When he told me about the additional diagnosis I felt happy and angry at the same time. After everything that had happened I was determined to investigate it myself, so I researched the condition. I did everything to try and get my head around the new information.

I was really worried about how Asha might cope with another 'condition'. It had already been six years of struggling to discover what was wrong with me and at least $6000 in expenses. I kept the Adult ADHD diagnosis from her for four weeks. I was anxious about how she was going to react to 'starting again', especially with new meds. I ended up telling her by opening up the chapter of a book to Adult ADHD Type 6, giving it to her and bolting. She read it and had to process it for a couple of days before we could even discuss it. It was not a happy time in the house. It brought up a lot of bad memories and once again we found ourselves revisiting a lot of things which were hard for both of us.

Dr Clarkson told me that often this type of thing can be genetic, so he encouraged me to get my parents to do an ADHD survey. They both have it. Mum returned a positive result for ADHD Type 2, 4 and 5. Dad was exactly the same as me – Type 6. Finding out about my parents actually made me feel better, as it helped them realise mental illness was real and they saw I was trying to help myself. It allowed us to have conversations about the illness and put it all out on the table.

RING OF FIRE

With both Asha and my family as support, I underwent a brain scan to confirm physiologically what the doctor had concluded through observation and consultation. Sure enough the brain scan confirmed ADHD and Bipolar II, and I saw what the doctor calls the 'ring of fire'. When my brain was relaxed, like when you watch a movie, imaging showed it with this ring of fire – it was wired and firing on all cylinders. When I'm playing a game of professional football or another highly stimulating activity, my brain is the opposite – it looks like a normal brain in a relaxed state.

When I saw it on the screen, I cried.

I couldn't shake the feeling that if everything so far had been wrong – wrong medication, wrong diagnosis, wrong solutions – why was life becoming a lot easier? Dr Clarkson believed that the reason things had got better for me was not solely because of the meds, but because I had moved out of inner city living and into a quiet, country lifestyle. I had removed many of the stimuli that triggered me and I had worked really hard to put boundaries in place.

It wasn't any picnic though. I still had to work exceptionally hard everyday to be normal; to try not to get back on the bottle and to stop the desire to go out. For me life had become a regimented and strictly controlled routine of coming home from work, taking work boots off, walking to fridge, cracking a can but limiting it to only two or three.

BATTLING GROG

I've spoken a lot in this book about my struggles with alcohol. I'm sure there's plenty of people reading it thinking why doesn't he stop drinking all together? Maybe that's the right thing to do, maybe not. It's not the right thing for me. With a whole heap of counselling and education about alcohol, I'm comfortable to have moderate amounts. Mind you, there is a step process I go through before alcohol touches my lips.

Step one is to ask myself the following questions: What mood am I in? What I mean by this is; why am I drinking? Am I emotional? Am I angry? Am I sad? Am I tired? Am I energised? Am I stressed? Has something gone wrong in my day?

Step two is what's my location? A safe location for me is at home or at a restaurant, a big risk is at a bar, in a nightclub at 5am, overseas, or in a football environment. The final step is who am I drinking with? Safe people include Asha, friends and family who understand my condition. A real risk for me is people who are confrontational, ex-players and people who want a piece of me.

If I have one cross in any of these steps then it's no alcohol for me. But if the perfect situation presented itself, I would feel comfortable to get drunk.

I've been working in the mining industry and that has helped to a point. There is zero tolerance to alcohol working in this sector and that set drinking boundaries for me. It scared me a little because once again I had an artificial external rule in place which was restricting my behaviour rather than taking control of it myself. Working the regular shift helped though, going to work every day. I'm not sure how the Fly In Fly Out guys do it, I know I'd find it hard to control the strict rules if I worked for one week on then was let off the leash for the other week.

CHASING THE STIMULUS

Looking back at my mood changes in the past when I've been drinking, I can see it all very clearly now. I'm having a good time, feel comfortable, feel safe, enjoying myself – then after the sixth beer, something just pops into me. Everything is heightened, like an intense feeling of blood flowing straight to my brain and I just can't cope – paranoia kicks in and irritability turns into aggression. It's all really stimulating, and to be honest it appeals to me; it makes me feel powerful, my body craves the stimulation. Once I get past that point it's like the tipping of the scales and then I start to chase the stimulus. It's what happened in my footy career. Footy was a massive stimulant and masked my ADHD and Bipolar II for all those years. I can see that far more clearly now.

Unfortunately it's not just grog that can tip the scales for me. In my unmedicated state I still want to chase the stimulus. There's lots of ways I do this: taking on too much work; trying to keep everyone happy to the detriment of myself and the ones I love; always saying yes. Some people think it's about approval, but it's not, it's about stimulus.

When I'm in this state I find I have racing thoughts, I eat more, I can never complete a task to its full potential and my energy levels are off the charts. I'm like a fly in a bottle, buzzing around, banging into things, never stopping, but never getting anywhere either.

It's the whole 'ring of fire' thing. When my brain is over-stimulated it's calm, when it's under stimulated it's clamouring for action.

The medication calms it down and stops my brain wanting to chase stimulus. It makes me extremely calm and able to work through volatile situations. I can see through it all now where previously I'd go down the drama queen route. It may sound silly to some, but now I can sit down and play Uno or watch a movie with my kids without getting up. For me the medication is like flicking a light switch on and off. My anger is gone, my impulsiveness has gone, the pain in my body from tensed up muscles – gone. I can get on a plane without a panic attack and, at last, I can sleep.

As well as new medication, I've changed my diet and I exercise a lot more. I'm on a 'blood diet' for O positive blood types – no wheat, no dairy, no caffeine – a 'hunter' diet. The benefits are really overwhelming and I feel better than I have felt for a long time.

MEDS, MEDS AND MORE MEDS

It's worth me reflecting a little on my efforts (and the efforts of the many medical professionals) to try and find the right medications. In 2009, when my world was going mad, I was on drugs for anxiety and depression, as well as testosterone for weight training. Boy that was a really bad combination for me, especially when you throw in alcohol on top of the manic behaviour.

After being diagnosed with Bipolar II, I went on a different drug which was in such small doses in retrospect it had more of a placebo effect. My doctor recently suggested I try a drug often prescribed to women for weight loss, but after I didn't sleep for two days, lost my appetite, and was countering the effects with anti-anxiety tablets, we knew that wasn't the solution.

The next attempt to find the right medication was a drug which targeted the temporal lobe of the brain, which is responsible for anger, pain and impulsive behaviour. The result of this drug was instant calmness, so that was good. I did also try a common ADHD drug used for kids but found after 10 days it just added fuel to the fire. I immediately became the man I was in Northbridge, I increased sports training by 20 per cent, didn't sleep, started to get the 'Superman feeling', felt I was hot shit. I really liked that feeling again, so I quickly rang the doctor and said *"Do you want me to spend time in jail or get better?"*. I recognised it straight away; that person in the mirror looking back at me, and pushed him away.

I've just started a trial of Dexamphetamine, and I'm very confident it will work. It's been very hard to get a prescription for it, and quite rightly so, it's sold for good money on the streets by drug-dealers. We'll wait and see, I suppose, but I hope it's a long term solution.

SEX AND RELATIONSHIPS

One area which has been affected by the medication and all the work with doctors is sex; but not in a bad way. Getting better mentally has revealed to me just how devoted I am to Asha.

During my football career I was unfaithful, and in Northbridge I would have classed myself as a sexual predator. I look back and see two reasons for this: I had a huge sex drive, which was helped by the fact that some women really get into that whole professional sportsmen thing. Secondly, I associated sex with the stimulation provided by the 'chase and kill' from a one night stand. I was devoid of any emotion during the chase, but afterwards I had a huge feeling of guilt because of the people I had inevitably betrayed.

I used to try and justify my behaviour to myself to get over the guilt, thinking things like I'm a young bloke and I need it. That sort of shit. When I started my relationship with Asha, I just continued that pattern. That's no excuse though. I loved Asha from the moment I met her, but it didn't stop me from being a total dickhead. I often think I would have liked to have met Asha 12 months later. As it was, when we did hook up, my wounds were still very much open – I was a woman-hater and for me it was all about getting revenge on previous relationships.

I've spoken publicly about what I call my 'werewolf' behaviour. Through certain periods when I was hyper manic, the full moon actually did something to me. I would get scared when I knew a full moon was due. My energy levels went up, I had no need for sleep, I would wander the streets, drink all day and not get drunk, and spend my nights in Northbridge strip clubs.

Now I'm back on track I'm so glad my relationship with Asha survived and we are now husband and wife. I'm compatible with Asha and she makes me feel good about myself in every way. There's no more guilt or game playing around sex, and no need for other females to boost my ego; my wandering eye has gone. It's what it should be, a normal bloke married to someone he loves.

CONTROLLING THE RAGE

I've reflected in this final chapter on the drinking, the womanising and all the other carry on, but what about my other massive challenge - anger?

I call it my Superman feeling; I'm invincible. It starts in my brain then flows through my body. I feel the blood fill my arms and fists and everything goes tense in my shoulders and forearms. It's easiest to describe as a colour – it's red – and I can see the red travelling through my body as I get angry.

Anger has always been the main emotion which has let me down and the first emotion to pop up in any scenario. As a kid, anger was always the solution in my household. If a problem couldn't be solved with angry words it could be solved physically with fists. Anger for me as an adult was often linked to grog. Whatever the trigger, the next step was to drink to calm anger, then anger would return tenfold, and then it would be on.

The AFL is very physical and aggressive. You had to be able to defend yourself on the ground, so I always had an outlet for anger when I played. The further I move away from that, the less I am on guard, and nowadays I am not so ready to engage in a fight. It's a bloody relief.

I still have some very volatile situations happening in my life but I haven't lost my temper once. Without doubt I think this is purely because of medication.

CLEARING THE DECKS

People may think I'm wealthy and asset rich and, yes, at the end of my AFL career and the height of my illness and manic behaviour, I had lots of money. I spent all of it on cars, houses, high-risk share portfolios, and entertaining all my 'friends'. I was always very generous, wanting to be liked and admired – always feeding the ego. I've subsequently found out this is linked very closely to both ADHD and Bipolar II.

It wasn't about people using me, it was me chasing the stimulation and the reward that was addictive – enough to keep doing it until I had nothing left. In fact, the day I had to give my Dad my 2003 Springer Softail Harley Davidson, my pride and joy, to repay a debt, I realised I'd gone broke.

It's been an upward struggle since then, with long stints of unemployment where I've needed Asha to support me, and lots of labouring, contract work and bloody hard yards to claw my way back. For 12 months I was doing 11-hour days earning $25 an hour flat rate. Being unemployed and then bringing in a low wage was humiliating for me as a man, a partner and a father. It is embarrassing to think that I had to buy a car for $2000, which was so beaten up it should have had a yellow sticker. I kept it for eight months because it was all I could afford. I'd pick up my kids from school in it and people would shake their heads... I could see them thinking "what has he done with his life?".

On that note I'm aware that people think I'm writing this book and going on the speaker circuit because I need the cash. I've seen the chat lines where people say it's fantastic what I'm doing bringing mental illness to the forefront, but the minute they hear about the book they lose respect. People seem to think there's a catch. In fact they are right, there is a catch. This book is a way of getting my message to a much wider audience and helping a lot more people. It may be clichéd but I'm more than ready to wear the criticism because I can only do so many talks, and this way I can get to more people. Also, some people aren't in the headspace where they're prepared to come to a talk or go public in anyway about these issues, so a book reaches those people as well.

So to those people who feel justified in questioning my motivation – go for it – I know why I'm doing this and that's all that matters.

Finally, as part of 'clearing the decks' I feel the need to make a comment about the state of mental health care in Australia.

I first looked for help in 2006 and it's now 2012 and I'm just emerging with the right solutions. A lot of God-awful things have happened in those six years and a lot of people have been hurt. What does that say about the mental health support network in Australia? I was fortunate enough to have a lot of contacts through the AFLPA which enabled me to jump queues to see professionals. Mind you, even jumping the queues saw my average waiting time around two weeks. Fame, or maybe it was notoriety, got me support which the average Joe Blow wouldn't be able to access.

Without my contacts what were my options? Turning up at an emergency ward and getting a shot of morphine? Or other options I did try, like drinking myself into oblivion or getting arrested and taking myself away from people I could hurt. If it wasn't for Dr John Clarkson taking a personal interest in me and ordering brain imaging, I would probably still be on the wrong medication.

FUTURE HORIZONS

Asha and I got married on New Year's Eve 2011 and we have moved back to Melbourne.

Living in south west Western Australia certainly served its purpose but we were isolated from family and friends and it had, in fact, turned into Groundhog Day. There was an opportunity to have a strong family network around us in Melbourne and a new job opportunity for me.

I am starting study to mentor elite athletes and I hope to do welfare work with the AFL helping other players. I also plan to travel around Australia and speak to people in the construction, mining and farming sectors to help men who relate to my story. I've started playing, as well as coaching, footy again, this time with my younger brother Dean at

Vermont Football Club in the Eastern Football League in Victoria. My dream job is to continue to work with the AFL, and men in general, to help people avoid the mistakes I have made.

My deep-lying passion, and the reason I am in the public arena, speaking to people, is that I believe my story may help prevent a suicide, or stop a person ending up in jail, or from hurting someone. It may stop someone from drink-driving and injuring themselves or someone else. Or it may simply stop the destruction of a relationship.

Already as a result of the Men in Black Ball and publicity associated with that, I have strangers messaging me, approaching me, stopping me in the shops, wanting to share their stories with me. There is a real need for this reaching out. It's much more prevalent than people would even start to suspect.

I'm not scared that I won't be able to cope with this; for me it is my therapy. I believe the journey will continue... I'm sure there's another book in it.

One thing that has become clear to me during this journey is that there is no end chapter. You may think you have the solution but, sure enough, there is always something else and another challenge to overcome.

I just want to help people get started. I'm not saying it's easy, it's bloody hard and it's ongoing, but let me leave you with this observation: before I came out and said I had a mental illness, I would attract aggressive people who wanted to have a go at me. That's disappeared. I now attract people who need help or just want someone to listen to them.

BLACK

I'd be bullshitting if I said it wasn't draining because it is, but I truly feel this is my purpose, my calling. I just have to do it.

CHAPTER 12
THROUGH THE EYES OF A LOVED ONE

Heath's wife Asha Montgomerie talks about her journey while Heath was struggling through his darkest days.

Too often we underestimate the power of a touch, a smile, a kind word, a listening ear, an honest compliment, or the smallest act of caring, all of which have the potential to turn a life around. - **Leo Buscaqlia**

I was raised in Roxby Downs, a remote mining town in South Australia. At the age of 14, I was sent to Loreto College in Adelaide, an all-girls, Catholic boarding school. I have a very loving and supportive family but it is safe to say that I learnt about loneliness at a very young age. It wasn't a bad lesson to learn, in fact, it has helped me face many confronting situations as an adult, none more so than with Heath.

MELBOURNE

I met Heath in the latter half of 2008, after he had just announced his retirement from the AFL. It was a Sunday afternoon and I was at College Lawn in Melbourne with my friend and room-mate, Jodie. We had just had a huge weekend and were busy debriefing on our shenanigans with a bottle of wine or two. Heath waltzed in with his arm in a sling and the other arm around a girl. We didn't take too much more notice of Heath and quietly sat in our corner, listening to the music and taking in the casual Sunday session atmosphere.

There seemed to be a lot of hype around Heath and his group of friends, which we didn't quite understand. It was approaching the end of the night and we were preparing to leave. We bumped into Heath and his friends on our way out and they seemed pretty happy to talk to us. We made small talk but I wasn't really showing any interest. After all, he had come in with a girl whom I assumed was his girlfriend. Heath told me he was an AFL footballer but I didn't believe him. I remember saying to him *"but you're too short"*. I thought that he was just trying to use it as a pick-up line. We swapped numbers but I never expected to hear from him again. I thought it was just an awkward yet polite way of saying goodbye. So I was very surprised to get a text from him 12 hours later asking if he could take me out on a date!

We arranged to catch up on the following Wednesday for dinner. I asked him to pick me up from my house – mainly because I couldn't remember what he looked like!

Yes, I was that drunk on the Sunday night. All I could remember was that he was short, had a grubby beard and I thought he was a 'wog'. I didn't even know his surname, so I couldn't Google him to see a photo. When he turned up at my door he was clean-shaven and I was pleasantly surprised by how attractive he was. The only thing I was right about was his height. The evening out was full of conversation and laughter. I was surprised by how much we had in common, including the fact that we were both still coming to terms with the end of our previous relationships. We started seeing each other and within a couple of months, Heath was flying to Melbourne more regularly to see me. I also found myself flying across the country to Perth to see him.

It was a simple relationship – we had fun when we saw each other and we didn't get too caught up in worrying about what the other one was doing when we weren't together. I still get butterflies in my stomach when I think back to our exciting Melbourne days. I was in a state of ignorant bliss. I was completely unaware of Heath's alter ego, who we now jokingly refer to as *Keith*. *Keith* had total disrespect for women and treated them like an animal he'd hunt down for sex. I never met *Keith* when I was in Melbourne. If I had, I would have run a mile before things got any more serious.

At the end of 2008, my job contract in Melbourne was nearing an end and I needed to decide where I would live. A job opportunity came up for me in Perth, so I jumped at the chance to be closer to Heath. I wasn't sure where the relationship was heading but I knew that I felt happy when I was around him and that was good enough for me. I have always jumped in head first with relationships – just ask my poor family and friends who used to sit back and shake their heads. Falling in love fast is my thing. This was certainly no different with Heath. I had two failed relationships to learn from and he was recovering from his failed marriage. I was convinced it was fate. What I didn't realise was that my move to Perth was the start of the most confronting, distressing and destructive 12 months for both of us.

We refer to our relationship in stages, Melbourne (2008), Northbridge (2009) and Bunbury (2010–11). I have already discussed our Melbourne relationship as ignorant bliss. In comparison, our Northbridge relationship was parasitic; we needed each other yet were draining each other at the same time.

NORTHBRIDGE

I first met Heath's alter-ego *Keith* at the start of 2009. Heath was playing football for St Mary's in Darwin and would fly out each weekend for the game. There was one trip in particular that played on my mind for a long time, which took place on the Australia Day long weekend. Heath was due to fly back to Perth after his game and we were going to watch the fireworks from my new workplace in the Perth CBD. He rang me extremely drunk. I could hear plenty of noise in the background – guys and girls. He was trying to tell me that it was a couple of guys having a quiet night. I couldn't believe that he was so blatantly lying to me. When I tried to call back, he had turned off his phone.

I had a sleepless night waiting for him to call. He never did. He called late the next day to tell me that he had missed his flight and he wouldn't be home until the next day. I spent the whole day worrying about what I had done wrong and wondering why he was behaving this way.

Then one Friday night, we planned to go out for drinks and stay at a hotel. When I arrived at the pub, Heath was already 10 beers in and flirting with the barmaid. I laughed it off because I didn't really know how else to respond. After about an hour, he just headed out of the bar. I followed him and he seemed surprised to see me – like he had forgotten that I was even with him. I decided to call it a night and was about to return to the room when he handed me his phone and said he just needed to run to get a kebab.

A 'sext message' appeared on his phone from a girl. I was mortified. I confronted him as soon as he got back with his kebab. He denied having any kind of relationship with this girl and insisted that she was a 'fuck' he had had not long after he'd split from his ex-wife. I could not find any sent items in his phone, so I accepted his explanation. I have never been a jealous person and have always given people the benefit of the doubt. Like any woman, I do not rate infidelity and will never understand it. I remember telling Heath that he should never feel trapped with me and should end things now if he wanted to be with other women. I knew it would be easier for me to deal with a relationship break-up rather than the deceit and humiliation of an affair.

In February 2009, we moved into a brand new apartment in Northbridge. I was looking forward to putting the 'Darwin' experience behind me. I didn't realise that it was an entrée for what was ahead; our Northbridge chapter. Honestly, I still struggle to put the pieces together of that year; it was an alcohol-fuelled roller coaster. Our lives revolved around always being out and about and we weren't necessarily fussy about the venue or atmosphere. We were both consuming large volumes of alcohol but each for very different reasons. While Heath was self-medicating for Bipolar II, I was drinking to escape the reality of life with *Keith*.

I wasn't stupid. As the year went on I discovered more text messages and guessed there were more hook-ups with girls Heath was hunting. He kept insisting that they were all before my time but I wasn't convinced. I became obsessed with checking Heath's mobile phone, which everyone knows is rule number one of what not to do in a relationship, but I felt so betrayed and needed evidence one way or the other. I kept telling myself that if I could just find just one text message that proved he had cheated, then that would be all the evidence I needed to find the strength to leave.

What was wrong with me? Why did I need more evidence than what I already had? He was staying out all night and not coming home. It's only now, two years down the track that I realise that there were at least seven separate nights through 2009 when he did not come home. One night I was trapped outside all night waiting for him to return with our key. I curled up near the back door and desperately tried to break the glass. I was freezing, scared and alone. He claims he slept on a park bench. On some of those nights he was locked up, other times I found multiple texts from women, and still other nights he just couldn't face me, so he walked the streets.

The question I now ask myself is why did I put up with all of this shit? It's hard to find a clear answer.

All of my insecurities culminated in a very dark way in August 2009. That was my rock bottom. It was the exact same time that Heath had started working with Lisa on the book; revealing to her his darkest secrets; finally telling someone the truth about his life.

Thinking back to that time makes me want to sob. I am still overwhelmed by the emotions I felt back then. One desperate late-night phone call to my parents around this time saw them jump on a plane from Port Lincoln to be with me. They arrived within 24 hours and didn't ask me any questions. They were upset and confused but even they could see that I was not able to explain my feelings. Heath was such a tosser, then. He told them that he thought I was upset with my hair and my nails. My parents got me through that time and were there when I needed them most.

My parents stayed with us for a week. While they were with us, Heath got locked up for public nuisance or drunk and disorderly… I can't remember which because his misdemeanours were all so close together in the later part of 2009. They're a bit of a blur. He had snuck out to the Hyde Park for a beer after my parents had gone to bed. They had no idea that he wasn't home until I got his phone call at 7am the next morning to ask me to pick him up from the police station. I didn't even care that he had been locked up and didn't respond at all. I told him that I didn't want to see him. A friend of Heath's phoned to say he would look after him for the day.

I went out for dinner that night with my parents at a friend's house. I welcomed the laughter and normality of a family dinner and realised how much I missed such simple things. While at dinner, I got another phone call to tell me Heath was very drunk and on his way home. We left our friends and I had no idea who or what we were going to find when we got home. Heath was too embarrassed to see my parents, so he asked me to get them out of the house so that he could sneak back upstairs and go to sleep … like no one would even know that he had been gone. My parents obliged him his request and said nothing. They had met *Keith* for the first time, in all his glory. They were extremely worried for me and I could see the despair on their faces.

I love them for not judging me at that time. I know that if they told me to leave him, I would have left. I would have let them pack my bags and I would have moved back with them to Port Lincoln. What they did say to me surprised me and gave me the strength to go on in my relationship with Heath. Dad cornered Heath the next day to have a talk, 'man to man', and find out *"what the bloody hell was going on with him"*. Without knowing the full extent of that conversation, I know that Dad asked Heath if he realised that he was destroying me while on his own path to self-destruction.

Mum had a similar talk with him and I think pleaded with him to consider me for a moment. It was the first time that Heath understood the impact that his actions and behaviour were having on me and I could see immediately the guilt and remorse on his face.

THE LONG ROAD TO RECOVERY

Over the next few days, Mum and Dad took me to see a hypnotherapist, a psychiatrist and a psychologist. All of them agreed that I was suffering from depression but that it was circumstantial due to the chaos of my life with Heath. None of them thought I needed medication. It was a relief to hear from professionals that I was not the one with the problem and that my depression would ease if my circumstances did.

I don't know what happened in hypnotherapy but I know that I started to feel better about myself. I felt brave enough to start dealing with my reality and I felt confident enough to put my foot down and start making some decisions for my own wellbeing. Once Mum and Dad felt comfortable that I was back on the right track, they flew back to Port Lincoln. As they left, they told me that despite what they had seen of Heath, they could see how genuine his love and compassion for me was, and they could see how much I loved him. They recognised that he needed help and they encouraged us both to help each other. It was OK to love Heath. Heath was a good man and I wasn't the only person who saw that. Thank you, Mum and Dad; that was the best advice ever.

So what happened between September and November of 2009? Heath writes about it in the first two chapters of this book.

I couldn't understand why it got worse during this period. I kept thinking, was it my fault? On top of whatever it was he was trying to deal with, was he now feeling guilty for ruining my life? I think so. I think he didn't know how to protect me from *Keith* but he was not prepared to lose me. He started to probe and question why he was behaving this way. He thought it was to do with the full moon, which is why he often refers to *"werewolf-like behaviour"* when he talks to the media. I think he used the full moon as an excuse for *Keith*, like a 'get out of jail free' card. I could deal with it because I could see how hard he was trying to be a better man.

After seeing so much of *Keith* in the early part of 2009, I was relieved to only have to deal with him for two days a month. I have heard many reporters ask Heath when did he realise he had a problem. If I could answer this on his behalf, I don't think he realised it at all until people pulled him up on it. He had to hear the opinion of strangers, who saw him as a thug, an alcoholic and a complete wanker. People didn't want to be associated with him. They didn't want to invite him to their weddings or parties. He got the sack from his job and tossed out of his business partnership. He was overlooked for everything.

I actually thank the media and the public for reacting the way they did. It convinced him to seek professional help and get the right diagnosis. It saved him, and it definitely saved our relationship.

A LIGHT APPEARS

In December 2009, Heath was diagnosed with Bipolar II and was given a script for Lithium… that beautiful little white pill. How remarkable, that such a small little tablet could make such a large difference to our lives.

After some desperate pleas to various people in the south west, Heath was offered a job as the league coach of Harvey Brunswick Leschenault Football Club (HBL). They welcomed us with open arms and we were both humbled by the support they showed when no one else wanted to know Heath. He threw himself in his coaching role and I saw a new pride grow in him. Health felt like he was helping people. He felt like he was being a good partner to me, and he was. We had a home for the first time and we both started to feel a little bit normal.

In mid-2010 Heath finally opened up to me about the time he was *Keith*; no holds barred. I remember feeling nauseous from the detail and brutal honesty. It was raw truth and the words poured from Heath's mouth like some form of exorcism. I had had my suspicions and questions beforehand, but, honestly, I had no idea of the extent of his behaviour.

I was dumb-founded that he was able to hide so many things from me and lie so easily when questioned. After the nausea subsided, feelings of isolation, betrayal and abandonment sunk in. The very core of our relationship, as I understood it, had been smashed against a wall and the same negative thoughts from the previous year swam through my head again; *"what the fuck?"..."how could he do this to me?"..."I don't deserve this"..."why me"..."is this my fault, somehow?"..."how do I start again?"..."where do I go?"..."how do I tell my family and friends?"..."how do I walk away from his kids?"..."how will I get through another separation?"*, and on and on.

I thought we were over. I did not believe that I could or would ever recover from that. Heath was admitting to be the man I feared and loathed – a chauvinistic, sex-crazed, arrogant cockhead. The tears did not stop for two days as I mourned the loss of Melbourne's 'ignorant bliss'.

During this exorcism, Heath admitted to juggling three other girls at the start of our relationship. I was crushed – for me and for the other girls. None of us deserved to be treated with such little respect. In a strange way, I was relieved to finally understand why a chunk of our relationship didn't quite fit together. It has taken me a long time to get over the exorcism of *Keith* and I would be lying if I said that I was completely over it now. I don't think I ever will be. It still pops into my mind from time to time, and has now become such an ever-present insecurity that I have sought counselling to try to overcome it.

I'm sure the million dollar question everyone is dying to ask is, why didn't I leave him? Simple – the desire to be with Heath was greater than the desire to leave him. I couldn't imagine my life without him, nor did I want a life without him. I agreed to go with him to visit clinical psychologist,

Helen Fowler. We spoke about the exorcism and Helen then gave me the most valuable advice. She said, *"Asha, you have obviously made a decision to stay with Heath or you wouldn't be here. Don't think about that decision or over analyse it, or you will go mad. Accept that you have decided to stay and feel good about that."* I think of Helen's words nearly every day and I am sure that I will use them as a way of thinking about many other parts of my life.

Once I got over my own reaction to the exorcism, I started to think about how Heath must be feeling about it all. He had exposed himself entirely to me and allowed himself to be utterly vulnerable, which was admirable and courageous. How many people could do this, knowing the possible consequences of such honesty? Heath started to keep a mood diary, which became a safe space for us both to understand his moods so that we could start to understand *Keith's* patterns. For the first time in our relationship, I was finding routine and calmness and a deeper connection with Heath. It was as if I had climbed into Pandora's Box with him and we were clawing our way out together.

Heath finally trusted that I truly loved him – not for Heath Black the ex-AFL footballer but for Heath Black, the man with Bipolar II and Adult ADHD who took me to hell and back.

Since changing medication in January 2010, I have rarely seen *Keith*. Don't get me wrong, *Keith* lives on in Heath somewhere and he can surface every now and then if we get complacent. The difference is that we both recognise *Keith's* red carpet entrance and we are usually able to meet him at the door and watch him until he is ready to leave again. I accept that *Keith* is a part of Heath but I am comfortable now that Heath has the upper hand.

Some might call this sweeping things under the carpet, which is another thing I am known to do, but this time that's just not the case. I acknowledge that Heath has a mental illness, which he can only control with medication. It is no different to a person who needs medication to control asthma or diabetes. Bipolar II and Adult ADHD are real illnesses with real physical and emotional side effects. They are not a convenient way to excuse bad behaviour, which is a common public misconception. People should not confuse people with Bipolar II and/or Adult ADHD with genuine arseholes with no excuses.

I am confident that our Northbridge experience will always be our relationship litmus test and all future issues will be compared to Northbridge. As far as I am concerned, we have had enough downs to help us appreciate the ups. If we could make it through Northbridge, we can make it through anything.

I would like to end my story by borrowing some powerful words from the poet Robert Frost:

> *"... Two roads diverged in a wood, and I –*
> *I took the one less travelled by,*
> *And that has made all the difference."*

Asha Montgomerie
November 2011

EPILOGUE

I spent a lot of time with Heath during the second half of 2009, interviewing him for this book. Having only just met him, I was unaware of just how precarious his life had become at that time. I listened to his stories without judgement not realising he was revealing to me things he had never spoken of before or even admitted to himself. The man he showed to me was brave, gentlemanly and conflicted, someone who was lost and desperately trying to find his way.

After his series of misdemeanours we decided to put this book on hold to allow him to work out what was going wrong in his life. He was diagnosed correctly with Bipolar II and Adult ADHD, after wrongly being treated for depression, and spent 2010 and 2011 getting back on track.

Writing *Black* has been a long process, but in that time I've seen a different man emerge to the one I started interviewing three years ago. A man who is willing to swallow his pride and face his own demons in the hope of helping others. A man who wants people to understand the contradictions and overwhelming difficulties associated with having a mental illness.

There are many men in Australia walking in Heath's shoes – maybe now they have voice.

Lisa Holland-McNair, 2012

ABOUT THE AUTHOR

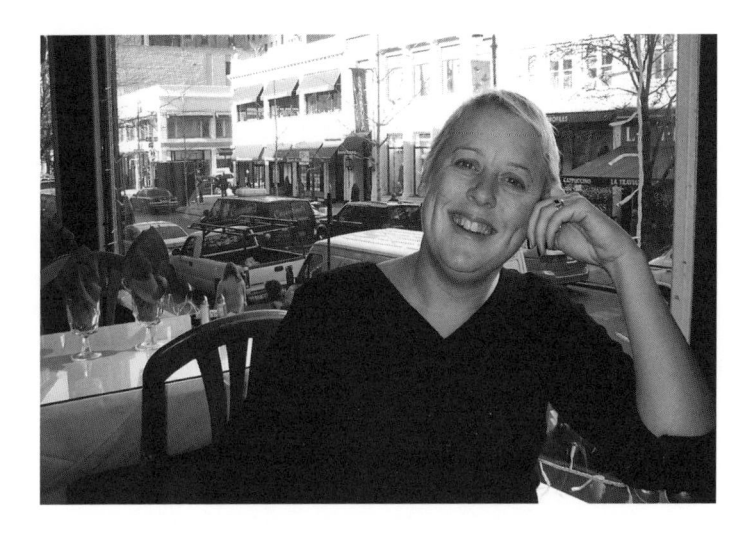

Lisa Holland-McNair specialises in writing non-fiction books and memoirs. She is the author of *Red Dust in Her Veins: Women of the Pilbara, Breaking New Ground: Stories of Mining and the Aboriginal People of the Pilbara; Who the Hell is Effie Crump?; and Make your Mark...The Graham (Polly) Farmer Foundation.* She has also had a short story published in *Short and Twisted 2007* as well as publishing her own children's book *Lola steals a plum* in 2011.

Lisa mainly writes about topical social issues and her aim is for the books to inform people and encourage robust debate in Australia. Some of the topics covered are Aboriginal Australians, challenges faced by men and women, mental illness and life in regional and remote Australia.

Lisa established Agenda Publishing in 2012 to publish books with social messages which help educate and inform people about what's happening in their community and country.

She lives in Perth, Western Australia with her husband Dean, and her two children, Drew and Amber.

www.hollandmcnair.com   **www.agendapublishing.com.au**